Pain Management in Cardiothoracic Surgery

Edited by
Glenn P. Gravlee, MD
Professor
Department of Anesthesia
The Bowman Gray School of Medicine;
Head, Section on Cardiothoracic Anesthesia
Wake Forest University Medical Center
Winston-Salem, North Carolina

Richard L. Rauck, MD
Assistant Professor
Department of Anesthesia
The Bowman Gray School of Medicine;
Director, Pain Control Center
Wake Forest University Medical Center
Winston-Salem, North Carolina

With 11 contributors

J. B. LIPPINCOTT COMPANY
Philadelphia

Pain Management in Cardiothoracic Surgery

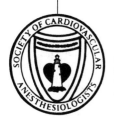

A Society of
Cardiovascular Anesthesiologists
Monograph

Acquisitions Editor: Mary K. Smith
Sponsoring Editor: Anne Geyer
Production Manager: Janet Greenwood
Production Services: Tage Publishing Service, Inc.
Compositor: Compset
Printer/Binder: R. R. Donnelley & Sons Company

6 5 4 3 2 1

Library of Congress Cataloging-in-Publication Data

Pain management in cardiothoracic surgery / edited by Glenn P. Gravlee, Richard L.
    Rauck : with an additional 11 contributors.
        p.   cm. — (A Society of Cardiovascular Anesthesiologists monograph)
    Includes bibliographical references and index.
    ISBN 0-397-51293-7
    1. Chest—Surgery—Complications.   2. Heart—Surgery—Complications.
3. Postoperative pain—Treatment.   I. Gravlee, Glenn P.   II. Rauck, Richard L.
III. Series.
    [DNLM: 1. Pain—therapy.   2. Postoperative Care.   3. Thoracic Surgery.
WF 980 P144 1993]
RD536.P35   1993
617.5′401—dc20
DNLM/DLC
for Library of Congress   92-48508
                                                                              CIP

The authors and publisher have exerted every effort to ensure that drug selection and dosage set forth in this text are in accord with current recommendations and practice at the time of publication. However, in view of ongoing research, changes in government regulations, and the constant flow of information relating to drug therapy and drug reactions, the reader is urged to check the package insert for each drug for any change in indications and dosage and for added warnings and precautions. This is particularly important when the recommended agent is a new or infrequently employed drug.

To Francis M. James III, whose guidance, support, patience, and teaching have enhanced our professional lives immeasurably.

Publication Committee of the
Society of Cardiovascular Anesthesiologists

Edward Lowenstein, MD, Chairman
Boston, Massachusetts

Frederick A. Burrows, MD
Toronto, Canada

Simon Gelman, MD, PhD
Boston, Massachusetts

Carl Lynch, III, MD
Charlottesville, Virginia

J. G. Reves, MD
Durham, North Carolina

T. E. Stanley, MD
Durham, North Carolina

David C. Warltier, MD
Milwaukee, Wisconsin

Contributors

James E. Brannon, MD
Assistant Clinical Professor of
  Anesthesiology
Medical College of Georgia
Acting Director
Division of Cardiothoracic
  Anesthesia and Critical Care
  Medicine
Georgia Baptist Medical Center
Atlanta, Georgia

F. Michael Ferrante, MD
Assistant Professor of Anaesthesia
Harvard Medical School
Director, Pain Treatment Service
Department of Anesthesia
Brigham and Women's Hospital
Boston, Massachusetts

Glenn P. Gravlee, MD
Professor
Department of Anesthesia
The Bowman Gray School of
  Medicine
Head, Section on Cardiothoracic
  Anesthesia
Wake Forest University Medical
  Center
Winston-Salem, North Carolina

Bernice R. Hecker, MD
Department of Anesthesia
Virginia Mason Clinic
Seattle, Washington

Kyle E. Jackson, MD
Assistant Professor
Department of Anesthesia
Wake Forest University Medical
  Center
Winston-Salem, North Carolina

P. Prithvi Raj, MD
National Pain Institute
Atlanta, Georgia

Richard L. Rauck, MD
Assistant Professor
Department of Anesthesia
The Bowman Gray School of
  Medicine
Director, Pain Control Center
Wake Forest University Medical
  Center
Winston-Salem, North Carolina

David A. Rosen, MD
Associate Professor
Departments of Anesthesia and
 Pediatrics
West Virginia University
Morgantown, West Virginia

Kathleen R. Rosen, MD
Associate Professor
Departments of Anesthesia and
 Pediatrics
West Virginia University
Morgantown, West Virginia

Kevin L. Speight, MD
Assistant Professor
Department of Anesthesia
Wake Forest University Medical
 Center
Winston-Salem, North Carolina

Gale E. Thompson, MD
Chairman
Department of Anesthesia
Virginia Mason Clinic
Seattle, Washington

Timothy R. VadeBoncouer, MD
Instructor in Anaesthesia
Harvard Medical School
Anesthesiologist
Brigham and Women's Hospital
Boston, Massachusetts

Richard L. Wolman, MD
Associate Professor
Department of Anesthesiology
Medical College of Virginia
Virginia Commonwealth University
Richmond, Virginia

Contents

Preface

Recent developments in the management of acute pain have revolutionized the postoperative care of surgical patients. Just a decade ago, intramuscular opioids constituted the only postoperative analgesic option available to most patients. In the interim, modalities such as patient-controlled analgesia, epidural or subarachnoid opiates, and interpleural local anesthetics have developed and grown. Therapeutic decisions that once were very simple have become remarkably complex. These changes, while clearly advancing patient care, impose additional burdens on physicians who counsel patients about, and subsequently implement, postoperative pain management. To deliver state-of-the-art postoperative analgesia, the clinician must be knowledgeable about current techniques, their advantages, disadvantages, and risks.

The nature of the patient population experiencing cardiothoracic surgery further complicates this picture. These patients tend to be at extremes of age and usually have advanced, life-threatening diseases. They undergo surgical procedures that intrinsically compromise cardiovascular and respiratory physiology, at least temporarily, and induce postoperative pain more severe than that associated with most other types of surgery. Much of the morbidity and mortality that ensue from these procedures occurs in the first few postoperative days, yet only recently has attention been directed toward improving clinical outcomes by altering postoperative pain management. Our purpose in developing this book was to provide a concise but thorough overview of pain mechanisms and management after cardiothoracic surgery. At two of the last three annual meetings of the Society of Cardiovascular Anesthesiologists, panels on this topic have generated large attendances and lively audience participation.

The chapter authors were advised to address the cardiothoracic surgical patient specifically, although this effort was sometimes compromised either by a relative paucity of literature specific to those patients, or by a propensity among investigators to combine abdominal and thoracic surgical patients into a single clinical group. We believe that the authors have competently reviewed the state of knowledge and placed complex issues in the best clinical perspective currently possible. The perceptive reader may yearn for more answers than the authors can provide, which reflects the nascent state of this discipline. We hope that some readers might be inspired to fill gaps in the state of knowledge by performing their own investigations.

Glenn P. Gravlee, MD
Richard L. Rauck, MD

Acknowledgments

We thank the Publications Committee of the Society of Cardiovascular Anesthesiologists for pursuing this idea for the annual monograph and for providing us with the opportunity to organize and edit it. Special thanks go to Terri Barkley and Barbara Baylor for adroitly handling correspondence, telephone communication, and some of the manuscript preparation. We are grateful to our departmental editor, Wilson Somerville, and to his assistants, Kim Barnes, Vicky Cranfill, and Addie Larimore, for their invaluable assistance with manuscript processing and editing. We greatly appreciate the time and care taken by the contributing authors despite their own busy schedules and the relentless deadline pressure we placed on them. Finally, we are indebted to Mary K. Smith and Anne Geyer of J. B. Lippincott Company for their patience, cooperation, and persistence.

Pain Management in Cardiothoracic Surgery

Pain Management in Cardiothoracic Surgery, edited by Gravlee and Rauck. J. B. Lippincott Company, Philadelphia © 1993.

F. Michael Ferrante
Timothy R. VadeBoncouer

1 | Epidural and Subarachnoid Analgesia for Thoracic Surgery

Since the introduction of epidural[1] and subarachnoid[2] opioids (collectively called "spinal opioids") in 1979, these modalities have become widely used for the management of postoperative pain. Their ease of administration and their relatively high benefit-to-risk ratio (analgesia with few side effects) make them ideal for the management of postoperative pain. Whether given as a single injection at the time of anesthesia, intermittent injections, or continuous infusions through indwelling epidural catheters, spinal opioids can provide intense and sustained pain relief.

EPIDURAL OPIOIDS

Mechanism of Action

Segmental analgesia (selective spinally mediated analgesia[3]) occurs through binding of opioids to receptors in the spinal cord.[4,5] The dorsal horn is richly populated with opioid receptors.

The grey matter of the spinal cord has a laminar cytoarchitectural organization. Lamina I (marginal layer) lies juxtaposed to the dorsal columns and Lissauer's tract. Lamina II has a gelatinous appearance from which its name is derived—the substantia gelatinosa. Lamina V contains the cell bodies of the spinothalamic tract neurons. Laminae

1

II, III and V are densely populated with opioid receptors. Segmental or spinal analgesia is achieved by binding of exogenously administered opioids to these opioid receptors.

Production of segmental analgesia requires a minimum concentration of opioid in the cerebrospinal fluid (CSF) and, by inference, in the dorsal horn of the spinal cord level mediating nociception. This is important to stress, because epidural opioids may produce analgesia via systemic absorption of opioids despite insignificant amounts of drug in the CSF. Suffice it to say that true segmental analgesia results from drug effects on the dorsal horn, with little or no contribution from systemic levels of opioid.

Lipid Solubility

The physicochemical property of lipid solubility best predicts the behavior of opioids as spinal analgesics. Although molecular weight,[6] molecular size,[6] and receptor binding affinity[7,8] certainly play a role, lipid solubility[4,9,10] determines the behavior of spinal opioids. Commonly used epidural opioids are listed in order of increasing lipid solubility in Table 1–1.

When an opioid is delivered to the epidural space, the drug may ultimately be cleared by several routes. Drug may bind to: (1) extradural fat,[4,7,14] (2) enter the epidural venous system and thus the systemic circulation,[4,9,15] (3) enter the posterior radicular spinal arteries and be delivered directly to the dorsal horn (Fig. 1–1),[4,16] or (4) penetrate the dura through diffusion across the arachnoid granulations and enter the CSF (see Fig. 1–1).[4,16]

Highly lipid-soluble drugs (e.g., fentanyl) are avidly absorbed by epidural fat and blood vessels.[4,7,14] Drug binding to epidural fat will decrease its availability for diffusion into the CSF. Such binding is unpredictable as epidural fat content varies widely among patients.

Diffusion of opioid into epidural veins will result in systemic opioid levels with attendant effects (Fig. 1–2). Substantial and prolonged entry into the circulation will result in supraspinal (systemic) rather than segmental (spinal) analgesia.

Uptake of opioid in spinal cord segmental arteries may rapidly deliver drug to the dorsal horn.[4,16] This feature may explain the rapid onset of analgesia along with the rapid transfer of drug across arachnoid granulations seen with highly lipid-soluble epidural opioids (Fig. 1–1).

TABLE 1-1. Dosage Regimens for Intermittent Administration of Epidural Opioids

Drug	Lipid Solubility[a]	Bolus Dose	Onset (min)	Duration (hours)	Comments
Morphine	1	2–5 mg	30–60	6–24	Due to spread in CSF, preferred for extensive incisions and when injection site is distant from source of nociception
Meperidine	30	50–100 mg	5–10	6–8	
Methadone	100	1–10 mg	10	6–10	May accumulate in blood with repetitive dosing[4,11,12]
Fentanyl	800	50–100 μg	5	4–6	Not recommended when incision is extensive or injection site is distant from source of nociception
Sufentanil	1500	10–60 μg	5	2–4	Higher doses may produce excessive sedation or ventilatory depression, presumably due to vascular uptake[13]

[a]Octanol/pH 7.4 buffer partition coefficient relative to morphine

Although dural transfer may or may not be increased as lipid solubility increases, it is at the very least inefficient for the highly lipophilic opioids because of the aforementioned factors. Hydrophilic drugs such as morphine may have more efficient dural transfer because they are not well absorbed by epidural fat or blood vessels.[6]

Once opioid has gained access to CSF, it may remain there or bind to spinal cord tissue. Sequestration of the drug in the CSF would be most likely to occur with the relatively lipid-insoluble (hydrophilic) opioids (i.e., morphine).[9,15,17,18] Accumulation of opioid in the CSF

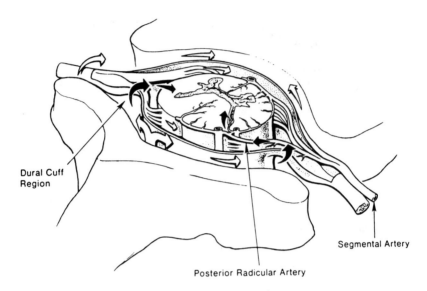

Dural Cuff Region

Segmental Artery

Posterior Radicular Artery

FIGURE 1–1.   Lipid-soluble epidural opioids may gain rapid access to the CSF by diffusion across the arachnoid granulations in the dural cuff region. The spread of opioids in the epidural space is denoted by white arrows. Spread within the CSF and spinal cord is depicted by black arrows. Lipid-soluble opioids may also be rapidly absorbed into the posterior radicular artery (a branch of the spinal segmental artery). Branches of the posterior radicular artery directly supply the dorsal horn. *(From Cousins and Bridenbaugh,*[4] *with permission.)*

leads to two well-recognized clinical features of spinal morphine: long duration of analgesia and predilection for cephalad flow within the CSF.[9,15,18]

Onset of Analgesia

Lipid-soluble agents quickly gain access to the dorsal horn via arachnoid granulations and spinal cord arterial blood flow resulting in rapid onset of analgesia (Fig. 1–1).[9,16,19] Although hydrophilic opioids transfer efficiently across the dura, they do so slowly and hence produce analgesia more slowly.[9,19]

Duration of Analgesia

Removal of opioid from the dorsal horn primarily occurs through local spinal cord blood flow. Highly lipid-soluble agents are rapidly absorbed into blood vessels from receptor sites, and analgesic duration is short.[4,9,16,19] Hydrophilic opioids, which preferentially distribute

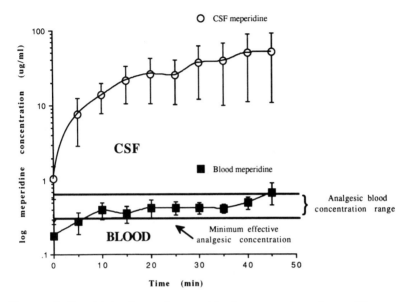

FIGURE 1–2.   CSF and central venous blood concentrations of meperidine (mean ± standard error) after epidural injection of 100 mg of meperidine (N = 8). (The minimum effective analgesic concentration (within the blood) and the range of analgesic blood concentrations were separately determined after intravenous injection of 100 mg meperidine.) Analgesia was related to CSF concentration in that patients having a high CSF/blood concentration ratio also had complete analgesia. The rapid rise in CSF meperidine concentration in the first 5 minutes after epidural injection also coincided with the onset of analgesia. For the majority of patients receiving epidural meperidine, the analgesic blood concentration range associated with intravenous injection (0.2–0.7 μg/ml) was achieved within 20 minutes. However, one patient never achieved an analgesic blood meperidine concentration at all during the study period, despite excellent analgesia. Thus, the major analgesic effect after epidural injection of a lipophilic opioid is spinally mediated, but vascular absorption may be significant. *(Data from Glynn et al.*[16]*)*

into the aqueous CSF milieu, diffuse poorly into blood vessels. Moreover, a depot of drug remains in the CSF for long periods with hydrophilic opioids thereby maintaining opioid receptor binding. Thus, analgesia is prolonged.[9,15,18,19]

Cephalad CSF Migration

The hydrophilic opioids, essentially sequestered in the CSF, are available to move cephalad via CSF bulk flow.[9,15,18,19] Analgesia is extended to include higher and higher dermatomes as successively more rostral concentrations of opioid are achieved.[15,20–26] Respiratory depression and vomiting may occur through direct interaction with centers in the medulla when significant concentrations of opioid reach the brain stem.

Lipid-soluble drugs are absorbed into lipids close to the site of injection and do not flow cephalad in the CSF to any significant degree.[4,7,14] Thus, opioid-related side effects are unlikely to be related to cephalad CSF drug movement. Side effects can occur with significant systemic levels of drug.

Table 1–1 and Figures 1–3 and 1–4 summarize the clinical characteristics of hydrophilic and lipophilic opioids following a single epidural injection.

Site of Injection

A general guideline for management of continuous epidural opioids (either single injection or infusion) is to place the catheter at the interspace crossed by the middle dermatome of the surgical incision. Spread of drug can occur both cephalad and caudad in such a manner as to optimize analgesia and minimize side effects. The highly lipid-soluble opioids are most dependent on catheter location for optimal segmental effect because of their limited ability to spread in the CSF.[27–32] The hydrophilic agents are much less dependent on injection site.[21–26]

Morphine administered in the lumbar epidural space can produce analgesia in dermatomes far removed from the initial site of injection.[21–26] Steidl and colleagues[24] compared the analgesic efficacy of thoracic and lumbar epidural morphine in postthoracotomy patients. Both groups obtained excellent analgesia while receiving identical low morphine doses. Some earlier studies did suggest that higher doses of morphine were required when injecting via the lumbar epidural space, at least in comparison to the doses required for lower abdominal and lower extremity analgesia. The onset time for thoracic dermatomal analgesia should also be delayed with lumbar epidural morphine as compared to thoracic epidural morphine.

Sjöström et al.[26] studied patients after major abdominal surgery. Patients were allowed to self-administer epidural morphine through a low thoracic or lumbar catheter (T10–L3). They achieved excellent pain relief from an average of only 0.5 mg/hr of morphine. Plasma morphine concentrations were well below those reported elsewhere for systemic (supraspinal) analgesia, indicating a spinally mediated

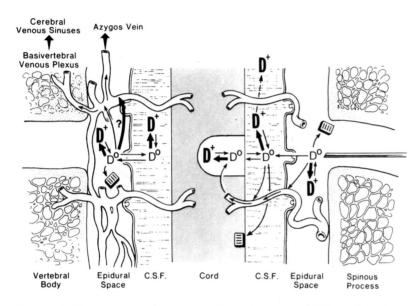

FIGURE 1–3.   Pharmacokinetic model for epidural injection of a hydrophilic opioid (morphine). D° = neutral form of drug able to diffuse through membranes; D^+ = ionized hydrophilic form of drug. After epidural injection of a highly ionized and hydrophilic opioid, only low concentrations of the lipid-soluble neutral form will be present in the epidural space. Thus, diffusion across the arachnoid granulations or into spinal arteries will be slow (slow onset of analgesia). Once within the CSF, most of the opioid will be present in the ionized form, thus presenting a small concentration gradient for diffusion to receptors in the cord or egress into blood vessels from occupied receptors (long duration of analgesia). The high concentration of ionized hydrophilic drug within the CSF will move rostrally with CSF flow (extension of analgesia over a wide number of dermatome). If significant concentrations of opioid reach the rostroventral medulla, nausea, vomiting and delayed respiratory depression may result. (*Modified from Cousins and Bridenbaugh,[4] with permission.*)

mechanism for pain relief. Excellent analgesia occurred despite catheter location near the caudad end of an extensive abdominal surgical incision.

Controversy exists as to the ability of the more lipid-soluble opioids to produce segmental spinal analgesia without significant supraspinal contribution. Bodily et al.[27] reported lower hourly fentanyl requirements and better pain scores in postthoracotomy patients receiving thoracic epidural fentanyl as compared to a group receiving lumbar epidural fentanyl. Badner and colleagues[28] were able to pro-

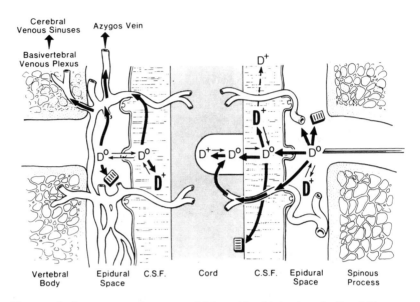

FIGURE 1–4. Pharmacokinetic model for epidural injection of a lipophilic opioid (e.g., meperidine or fentanyl). D^o = neutral form of drug able to diffuse through membranes; D^+ = ionized hydrophilic form of drug. After epidural injection of a mostly ionized lipophilic opioid, low concentrations of the neutral form will rapidly diffuse through the arachnoid granulations into CSF, into spinal radicular arteries and thereby to the dorsal horn, and into epidural veins (rapid onset of analgesia). Because of brisk spinal artery flow and slow epidural venous flow, transfer of drug to the spinal cord will occur while the concentration gradient is high (rapid onset of analgesia). Significant vascular absorption into epidural veins will rapidly reduce the concentration gradient (short duration of analgesia, potential early respiratory depression). Diffusion of opioid from receptors into the venous system will be equally as rapid (short duration of analgesia, potential early respiratory depression). As these opioids are lipophilic, there will be significant binding to fat and other nonspecific (nonreceptor) sites. For all the aforementioned reasons, the amount of ionized species (D^+) available to flow rostrally in the CSF will be insignificant (no potential for delayed respiratory depression). *(Modified from Cousins and Bridenbaugh,[+] with permission.)*

vide analgesia after thoracotomy by utilizing lumbar epidural fentanyl infusions. However, when patients had the best pain relief, systemic fentanyl levels were within the range reported for systemic analgesia. Another study reported successful thoracic analgesia when large doses (200 µg) of fentanyl were given through a lumbar epidural catheter every 3 to 4 hours.[29] The authors reported an alarmingly high incidence of sedation (90%) after each dose. Unfortunately, systemic fentanyl levels were not measured.

The controversy over the utility of epidural fentanyl for segmental analgesia has been recently extended to include other situations, in particular those in which the surgical incision is small and/or the catheter location along the neuraxis is close to the spinal cord segments receiving nociceptive input. Estok et al.[30] compared patient-controlled intravenous fentanyl to patient-controlled lumbar epidural fentanyl for treatment of pain after abdominal or lower extremity surgery using a double-blind crossover protocol. The two groups had comparable pain relief and plasma fentanyl levels during therapy. A similar result was noted in another study comparing infusions of intravenous and epidural fentanyl for analgesia after cesarean delivery.[31] Quality of analgesia, plasma fentanyl levels, and incidence of side effects were similar in both groups by the 12th hour of therapy. Last, Loper and colleagues compared continuous infusions of intravenous and epidural fentanyl for treating the pain of knee arthrotomy using a double-blind protocol.[32] They also found no differences in pain scores or systemic fentanyl levels between the two groups.

Clearly, the use of lumbar epidural fentanyl (and by inference all highly lipid-soluble opioids) cannot be recommended for the treatment of upper abdominal and thoracic pain.[27,29] High systemic fentanyl levels may result.[28,31,32] Pain relief is incomplete, and this technique appears to have no advantages over intravenous fentanyl.[31,32] Lipid-soluble drugs have limited ability to spread in the CSF and thus may not reach the appropriate spinal cord levels to produce analgesia.[4,7,14] Epidural fentanyl is probably best used with a thoracic epidural catheter for upper abdominal and thoracic pain.

Bolus Versus Continuous Infusion

Epidural opioids can be delivered as intermittent injections or continuous epidural infusions. As no special equipment is required, intermittent injection therapy is technically simpler. The long duration of action of morphine makes it the ideal agent for intermittent injection as the need for reinjection is infrequent.[33,34] Smaller doses of morphine should be administered initially in order to determine a reliable analgesic dose associated with few side effects. Small dose increments can be given if the initial dose is inadequate. Ready and colleagues have effectively employed this technique by permitting nursing staff to reinject epidural opioids when pain recurs.[35] Obviously, extensive nursing education is required.

Lipid-soluble opioids have much shorter durations of action than morphine when administered by intermittent injection; thus lipid-soluble opioids require frequent reinjection.[4,9,16,19] When extended pain relief is desired, these agents can be given as a continuous epidural infusion in an attempt to minimize the need for reinjection (Table 1–2).[28,31,32,38–41]

Continuous infusions of epidural morphine have also been used.[42,43] As a single initial injection of 4–5 mg of morphine may produce prolonged analgesia,[44] infusion rates should be low. Higher rates may be associated with increased risk of delayed side effects because this agent may accumulate and migrate rostrally in the CSF. Suffice it to say that because of its low lipid solubility, if an intermittent injection technique is chosen, epidural morphine represents the best choice.

Irrespective of administration by intermittent injection or continuous infusion, it is prudent to give smaller doses than ordinarily administered through a lumbar catheter when morphine is used via a thoracic catheter. Although opioid can reach the brain stem in either case, greater concentrations of morphine may reach the brain stem sooner if excessive doses are given in the thoracic area.[45]

TABLE 1–2. Epidural Opioid Infusions

Drug	Usual Infusion Rate (mg/hr)	Comments
Morphine	0.2–1.0	Lowest effective infusion rates should be used after a small bolus
Meperidine	10–25	Prolonged therapy may result in accumulation of normeperidine with risk of myoclonus and seizures[36,37]
Fentanyl	0.03–0.1	Contribution of systemic level to analgesia may be significant[31,32]

SUBARACHNOID OPIOIDS

The previous discussions have focused primarily on epidural administration of opioids. Epidural administration is preferred when protracted postoperative analgesia is desired as indwelling epidural catheters permit continuous or repeated opioid therapy. Direct instillation of opioid into the CSF (subarachnoid delivery) also produces potent analgesia.[2,3,18,46] Segmental analgesia via subarachnoid administration requires smaller doses than epidural administration.[18,47,48] As drug is delivered directly to the CSF, competition for drug absorption by epidural fat and blood vessels is avoided.[18,49] Onset of analgesia is usually faster.[49]

Most other factors determining the clinical actions of subarachnoid opioids are as previously described for epidural opioids, except for the slightly faster onset times. As with epidural administration, lipid solubility is paramount in determining extent and duration of analgesia.[7,10,50] As postoperative use of indwelling subarachnoid catheters is not clinically popular, only subarachnoid morphine will reliably produce sustained pain relief from a single injection. Subarachnoid morphine may produce analgesia of up to 24 hours duration, as with epidural morphine administration.[47,48,50,51]

Most clinical experience with subarachnoid opioids has been with morphine. Doses of 0.25–1.0 mg produce reliable, long-lasting analgesia.[46–52] These doses are about one fifth that of effective epidural morphine doses. This indicates a fairly reliable dural transfer fraction of 20% when morphine is administered epidurally. Due to competitive binding with fat, blood vessels, and nonspecific binding sites, reliable dural transfer fractions for the lipid-soluble opioids are difficult to predict.[53] Moreover, nonspecific binding of lipid-soluble opioids to fatty fiber tracts of the spinal cord may make even direct subarachnoid dose requirements of these agents uncertain.[17] A wide range of subarachnoid fentanyl doses (6.25–50 μg) will provide similar degrees of analgesia.[54]

Subarachnoid opioids are usually given as a single injection during administration of spinal anesthesia for surgery. Thus, extension of analgesia beyond the usual duration of action of the drug will require repetitive dural puncture. Morphine is therefore the subarachnoid opioid of choice for prolonged postoperative pain management.[47,48,50,51]

Table 1–3 summarizes commonly used dosing regimens for subarachnoid administration of opioids.

TABLE 1–3. Dosage Regimens for Subarachnoid Opioids

Drug	Dose	Onset (min)	Duration (hours)	Comments
Morphine	0.1–0.75 mg	15–30	10–30	Doses greater than 0.5 mg may produce high incidence of side effects[55-57]
Meperidine	10–30 mg	5	10–30	High doses have been employed for surgical anesthesia[58]
Fentanyl	10–50 μg	5	4–6	Higher doses will not prolong or intensify analgesia but may substantially increase side effects

SIDE EFFECTS OF SPINAL OPIOIDS

The incidence of side effects is probably no different between the epidural and subarachnoid routes of administration when reasonable doses are employed.[59]

Respiratory Depression

Respiratory depression is the most feared side effect of spinal opioid therapy and certainly the most potentially threatening to the patient. Respiratory depression occurs as a result of drug delivery to the respiratory control centers located in the brain stem. Delivery occurs via: (1) cephalad migration in CSF bulk flow, and/or (2) absorption into the circulation and subsequent delivery via cerebral blood flow. Following a single epidural[9,60-62] or subarachnoid injection,[10,63-65] the former mechanism results in delayed respiratory depression and the latter in early respiratory depression.[4,9,10,45] The "delay" occurs as a result of the time necessary for opioid to ascend in the CSF and interact with brain stem opioid receptors in the respiratory center.

Both lipid-soluble and hydrophilic agents can produce an early phase of respiratory depression (within 2 hours) after a single injection of spinal opioid.[4,9,10,45] The mechanism is no different from that observed following a parenteral injection of the same opioid: vascular uptake of drug and subsequent systemic delivery to the brain.[66] After this early phase, the lipid-soluble drugs are usually without further respiratory effect, reflecting their limited tendency to migrate cephalad in the CSF. Morphine, with its poor lipid solubility, is the prototypical agent producing delayed respiratory depression.[60-62] This effect may persist for up to 24 hours after the initial dose.[66]

The incidence of respiratory depression following spinal opioid administration is unknown. This is probably a reflection of the widely different criteria employed to define its occurrence. A decrease in respiratory rate (usually below 8 to 10 breaths per minute) is most commonly employed to denote the presence of respiratory depression. Ready has argued that respiratory rate alone is an unreliable predictor of changes in respiratory drive during spinal opioid therapy.[35,66] Similarly, changes in arterial pCO_2 and tidal volume may not accurately predict the presence of respiratory depression.[35] These uncertainties have led to a lack of consistent monitoring standards for patients receiving spinal opioids.

Given the uncertainties surrounding the parameters used to define respiratory depression, mild elevations of arterial pCO_2 (45–50 mm Hg) or modest declines in respiratory rate (8–10 breaths per minute) in otherwise healthy patients require no intervention other than continued observation. Immediate treatment is indicated when changes are severe. Naloxone will specifically reverse the respiratory effects of spinal opioids and may be lifesaving. In an apneic patient, an intravenous dose of 0.4 mg usually restores spontaneous ventilation. If respiratory depression is less severe (e.g., 4–8 breaths per minute), small increments of naloxone (0.04 mg) can be given. In either case, repeated doses of naloxone may be necessary due to its short half-life,[67] or a continuous intravenous infusion may be started (5 μg/kg/hr).[68] If respiratory depression requires naloxone for treatment, the patient should be observed in a monitored setting (intermediate care or intensive care unit).

The concomitant effects of naloxone administration on analgesia have been incompletely studied. Naloxone infusions of 5 μg/kg/hr have not affected the quality of epidural morphine analgesia while being sufficient to reverse respiratory depression.[68] An infusion rate of 10 μg/kg/hr has been shown to affect the duration of epidural morphine analgesia after intermittent injection.[68] Infusion rates of both 5 and 10 μg/kg/hr have been shown to reverse respiratory depression and affect the quality of analgesia in patients receiving epidural fentanyl.[69]

Nausea

Nausea and/or vomiting are caused by cephalad flow of opioid in CSF[70] or systemic transport[71-73] of significant opioid levels to the vomiting center and the chemoreceptor trigger zone in the medulla. The actual incidence of nausea is unknown. An early report by Bromage documented a 50% incidence of nausea or vomiting in human volunteers after epidural injection of morphine.[70] Ready more recently reported an incidence of 29% in postoperative patients receiving intermittent injections of epidural morphine.[74] The epidural use of lipid-soluble opioids, however, is believed to be associated with a greatly reduced incidence of nausea and vomiting.[71-73]

Nausea can be effectively treated with conventional antiemetics. Recently, transdermal scopolamine has been shown to be effective in reducing the incidence of nausea after epidural morphine.[75,76] This therapy is most effective when administered for 8 to 12 hours preceding epidural morphine.

Intravenous (i.v.) naloxone can be used when nausea is severe or prolonged. Small incremental doses of naloxone (0.04–0.1 mg) are administered in an attempt to preserve analgesia (especially with lipid-soluble opioids). Such practice is theoretically sound as CSF opioid concentrations in the brain stem are presumably much lower than at the site of administration. Thus, nausea may be more easily antagonized with small doses of naloxone. If nausea continues, an intravenous naloxone infusion can be implemented (1 µg/kg/hr, and "titrate" rate to effect).

Low doses of the agonist–antagonist drugs butorphanol[77,78] (0.25–0.5 mg i.v.) or nalbuphine[79,80] (1–3 mg i.v.) may also reverse nausea and other µ-receptor effects (i.e., nausea, pruritus, respiratory depression, etc.).

Pruritus

Although quite common with morphine, spinal opioid-induced pruritus is rarely severe and rarely requires treatment.[81] The possible spinal cord mechanisms involved in the production of spinal opioid-induced pruritus have been reviewed by Balantyne et al.[82] Histamine plays a negligible role in the production of spinal opioid-induced pruritus.[82]

Despite the negligible role of histamine in the pathogenesis of pruritus, antihistaminics can be used to treat mild pruritus. Severe itching may require incremental intravenous naloxone therapy as described earlier.

Urinary Retention

The mechanisms for spinal opioid-mediated urinary retention have been elegantly elucidated by Durant and Yaksh.[83] Subarachnoid morphine inhibits volume-induced bladder contractions and blocks the vesico–somatic reflex necessary for external sphincter relaxation.[83]

Bladder catheterization may be required in patients receiving spinal opioids. Naloxone administration may also be effective, but dose requirements may be so high as to reverse analgesia. A more desirable drug treatment for urinary retention is obviously needed. Spinal opioid-mediated urinary dysfunction may be attenuated by β-adrenergic and dopaminergic agonists, and α-adrenergic antagonists as reported in recent animal studies.[83] Validation in human subjects awaits further research.

Inhibition of Gastrointestinal Function

In volunteers receiving lumbar epidural morphine, Thorén et al. reported delayed gastric emptying as well as delayed orocecal and small intestinal transit times.[84] In patients following abdominal surgery, however, systemic opioid use resulted in a greater decrease in gastric emptying than spinal opioids, despite provision of equivalent analgesia.[85] It has been hypothesized that spinal cord mechanisms are involved in impaired gastrointestinal function after spinal opioid therapy.[86,87] Spinal opioids may thus delay postoperative recovery of bowel function.[84–87] It should be emphasized, however, that equivalent analgesia with parenteral opioids may result in even greater delay.

Conclusion

In summary, the single physiochemical property that best predicts the behavior of both epidural and subarachnoid opioids as spinal analgesics is lipid solubility. Hydrophilic opioids have a long onset of action but a prolonged duration of analgesia. Lipophilic opioids give quick but relatively short-lived pain relief. Thus, hydrophilic opioids are essentially sequestered in the CSF, explaining their propensity to give rise to late respiratory depression. Lipophilic opioids preferentially cause early respiratory depression due to elevated systemic blood levels of drug. Pruritis, nausea, and urinary retention are also caused by administration of both epidural and subarachnoid opioids. The incidence of side effects is probably no different when the two routes of administration are compared. In short, the use of spinal opioids has a high benefit-to-risk ratio causing profound analgesia with a relatively low incidence of side effects.

Appendix

Epidural Clonidine

RICHARD L. RAUCK

Many nonopiate analgesics are being investigated for acute post surgical pain, a result of recent investigations identifying nonopiate dependent anatomic pathways and pharmacologic receptors. Much of this work is focused at the spinal cord level where first order afferent neurons synapse in the dorsal horn of the spinal cord. Modulation of pain either through ascending or descending pathways can be augmented pharmacologically. The inability of some patients to achieve postoperative analgesia with spinal opiates probably reflects the potentially dominant role of these nonopiate algesic pathways. The use of nonopiate analgesic agents for these patients would allow pain relief postoperatively.

Theoretically, an advantage to nonopiate analgesics relates to the side effects of opiates. Nonopiates do not appear to have many of the side effects or risks of opiates including respiratory depression, urinary retention, nausea and vomiting, or pruritus. Unfortunately, ideal agents do not yet exist and nonopiates possess their own side effect profiles that can preclude their effective use.

Of the different classes being investigated, the alpha-II agonists have witnessed the most extensive use clinically. Clonidine, the most widely studied alpha-II agonist, has had the necessary and appropriate spinal cord toxicity studies performed to safely allow its spinal cord administration in humans.[88,89] Multiple clinical studies have demonstrated its analgesic efficacy in the postoperative period.[90-92] Some work has questioned whether the analgesic effect of clonidine is spinal cord mediated or secondary to systemic redistribution[93]; other studies refute this.[90-92] This discrepancy may exist, in part, because of different doses employed. Small doses may not be sufficient in all patients postoperatively.

Clonidine has been studied in the postoperative period for thoracic surgery. In a double-blind randomized study, Gordh reported 20 patients undergoing thoracotomy. Ten patients received clonidine 3 ug/kg epidurally and a control group (n = 10) received epidural saline postoperatively.[94] The clonidine group demonstrated no difference in PCA pethidine use when compared to the control group, and pain scores were similar between groups. Petit studied 30 patients undergoing laparotomy and right thoracotomy for esophagogastrectomy who received epidural clonidine 2 ug/kg (n = 10), epidural MSO_4, 50 ug/kg (n = 10), or other combination of epidural MSO_4 and clonidine (n = 10).[95] Significant pain relief was found for all groups. The combination of MSO_4 and clonidine in this study potentiated the intensity but not the duration of pain relief seen with either epidural morphine or epidural clonidine. The difference between these studies is unclear. Some authors have suggested that higher doses of clonidine will produce significantly greater analgesia than lower doses. Also, clonidine has been shown to potentiate morphine in nonthoracic surgical cases. This effect is synergistic and may not be present when clonidine is administered as the sole agent.

Alpha-II agonists will undoubtedly not replace the opiates as primary analgesics for posthoracotomy patients. However, thoracotomies represent a very pain-intensive procedure, and work by Stenseth et al. demonstrated in a single dose design that opiates (MSO_4) would achieve analgesia in only 73% of these patients.[96] Repeating the dose of opiate will result in improved analgesia in some of the patients but a subset of patients will not receive significant analgesia, reflecting the multiple pathways for afferent pain input. Local anesthetics represent an option for some of these patients but their risks can make them undesirable. Alpha-II agonists will provide a valuable adjunct role in these patients and can assume a primary role for patients in whom narcotics are contraindicated.

The side effects and risks of clonidine must be considered prior to use. Hypotension appears more frequently after small or medium boluses. Large boluses will provide significant alpha-I agonist peripheral effects to maintain blood pressure, and the use of continuous infusions (e.g. −20 ug/hr) has avoided significant hypotensive effects. Sedation often results after large boluses, although respiratory depression has not been observed except in combination with epidural morphine. Dry mouth can result with prolonged use but has not been a problem with postoperative patients.

The search for analgesic agents devoid of side effects and risks will continue in the future. For the present, most will continue utilizing opiates as first-line epidural agents for most thoracic surgery. The combination of different classes of agents will allow tailoring of analgesic needs to the individual patient condition.

References

1. Behar M, Magora F, Olshwang D, Davison JT: Epidural morphine in the treatment of pain. Lancet i:527, 1979
2. Wang JK, Nauss LA, Thomas JE: Pain relief by intrathecally applied morphine in man. Anesthesiology 50:149, 1979
3. Cousins MJ, Mather LE, Glynn CJ et al: Selective spinal analgesia. Lancet i:1141, 1979
4. Cousins MJ, Cherry DA, Gourlay GK: Acute and chronic pain: Use of spinal opioids, p. 955. In Cousins MJ, Bridenbaugh PO (eds): Neural Blockade in Clinical Anesthesia and Management of Pain, 2nd ed. Philadelphia, Lippincott, 1988
5. Yaksh TL, Noveihed R: The physiology and pharmacology of spinal opiates. Ann Rev Pharmacol Toxicol 25:443, 1975
6. Moore RA, Bullingham RES, McQuay HJ et al: Dural permeability to narcotics: In vitro determination and application to extradural administration. Br J Anaesth 54:1117, 1982
7. Mather LE: Clinical pharmacokinetics of fentanyl and its newer derivatives. Clin Pharmacokinet 8:422, 1983
8. Freye E: The mode of action of opioids. In: Opioid Agonists Antagonists and Mixed Narcotic Analgesics. Theoretical Background and Considerations for Practical Use, p. 15. Berlin, Springer-Verlag, 1987
9. Sjöström S, Hartvig P, Persson MP, Tamsen A: Pharmacokinetics of epidural morphine and meperidine in humans. Anesthesiology 67:877, 1987
10. Sjöström S, Tamsen A, Persson MP, Hartvig P: Pharmacokinetics of intrathecal morphine and meperidine in humans. Anesthesiology 67:889, 1987
11. Gourlay GK, Wilson PR, Glynn CJ: Pharmacodynamics and pharmacokinetics of methadone during the perioperative period. Anesthesiology 57:458, 1982
12. Gourlay GK, Willis RJ, Wilson PR: Postoperative pain control with methadone: influence of supplementary methadone doses and blood concentration-response relationships. Anesthesiology 61:19, 1984
13. Cohen SE, Tan S, White PF: Sufentanil analgesia following cesarean sec-

tion: Epidural versus intravenous administration. Anesthesiology 68:129, 1988

14. Andersen HB, Christensen CB, Findlay JW, Jansen JA: Pharmacokinetics of epidural morphine and fentanyl in the goat, abstracted. Pain 19:A564, 1984

15. Gourlay GK, Cherry DA, Cousins MJ: Cephalad migration of morphine in CSF following lumbar epidural administration in patients with cancer pain. Pain 23:317, 1985

16. Glynn CJ, Mather LE, Cousins MJ et al: Peridural meperidine in humans: Analgetic response, pharmacokinetics and transmission into CSF. Anesthesiology 55:520, 1981

17. Dickenson AH, Sullivan AF, McQuay HJ: Intrathecal etorphine, fentanyl, and buprenorphine on spinal nociceptive neurones in the rat. Pain 42:227, 1990

18. Nordberg G: Pharmacokinetic aspects of spinal morphine analgesia. Acta Anaesthesiol Scand 79:1, 1984

19. Tamsen A, Sjöström S, Hartvig P et al: CSF and plasma kinetics of morphine and meperidine after epidural administration, abstracted. 59: A196, 1983

20. Nordberg G, Hedner T, Mellstrand T, Dahlström B: Pharmacokinetic aspects of epidural morphine analgesia. Anesthesiology 58:545, 1983

21. Larsen VH, Iversen AP, Christensen P et al: Postoperative pain treatment after upper abdominal surgery with epidural morphine at thoracic or lumbar level. Acta Anaesthesiol Scand 29:566, 1985

22. Niv D, Rudick V, Golan A, Cháyen MS: Augmentation of bupivacaine analgesia in labor by epidural morphine. Obstet Gynecol 67:206, 1986

23. Jensen PJ, Siem-Jorgensen P, Nielsen TB et al: Epidural morphine by the caudal route for postoperative pain relief. Acta Anaesthesiol Scand 26:511, 1982

24. Fromme GA, Steidl LJ, Danielson DR: Comparison of lumbar and thoracic epidural morphine for relief of postthoracotomy pain. Anesth Analg 64:454, 1985

25. Sullivan SP, Cherry DA: Pain from an invasive facial tumor relieved by lumbar epidural morphine. Anesth Analg 66:777, 1987

26. Sjöström S, Hartvig D, Tamsen A: Patient-controlled analgesia with extradural morphine or pethidine. Br J Anaesth 60:358, 1988

27. Bodily MN, Chamberlain DP, Ramsey DH, Olsson GL: Lumbar versus thoracic epidural catheter for post-thoracotomy analgesia, abstracted. Anesthesiology 7:A1146, 1989

28. Badner NH, Sandler AN, Colmenares ME: Lumbar epidural fentanyl infusions for post-thoracotomy patients, abstracted. Anesthesiology 71:A667, 1989

29. Melendez JA, Cirella VN, Delphin ES: Lumbar epidural fentanyl analgesia after thoracic surgery. J Cardiothorac Vasc Anesth 3:150–153, 1989

30. Estok PM, Glass PSA, Goldberg JS et al: Use of patient-controlled analgesia to compare intravenous to epidural administration of fentanyl in the postoperative patient, abstracted. Anesthesiology 67:A230, 1987

31. Ellis DJ, Millar WL, Reisner LS: A randomized double-blind comparison of epidural versus intravenous fentanyl infusion for analgesia after cesarean section. Anesthesiology 72:981, 1990

32. Loper KA, Ready LB, Downey M et al: Epidural and intravenous fentanyl infusions are clinically equivalent after knee surgery. Anesth Analg 70:72, 1990
33. Modig J, Paalzow L: A comparison of epidural morphine and epidural bupivacaine for postoperative pain relief. Acta Anaesthesiol Scand 25:437, 1981
34. Rawal N, Sjöstrand UH, Dahlström B et al: Epidural morphine for postoperative pain relief: A comparative study with intramuscular narcotic and intercostal nerve block. Anesth Analg 61:93, 1982
35. Ready LB, Oden R, Chadwick HS et al: Development of an anesthesiology-based postoperative pain management service. Anesthesiology 68:100, 1988
36. Hershey LA: Meperidine and central neurotoxicity. Ann Intern Med 98:548, 1983
37. Armstrong PJ, Bersten A: Normeperidine toxicity. Anesth Analg 65:536, 1986
38. Welchew EA, Thornton JA: Continuous thoracic epidural fentanyl. Anaesthesia 37:309, 1982
39. Bailey PW, Smith BE: Continuous epidural infusion of fentanyl for postoperative analgesia. Anaesthesia 35:1002, 1980
40. Boudrenult D, Brasseur L, Samii K, Lemoing JP: Comparison of continuous epidural bupivacaine infusion plus either continuous epidural infusion patient-controlled epidural injection of fentanyl for postoperative analgesia. Anesth Analg 73:132, 1991
41. Chien BB, Burke RG, Hunter DJ: An extensive experience with postoperative pain relief using postoperative fentanyl infusion. Arch Surg 126:692, 1991
42. El-Baz NM, Faber LP, Jensik RJ: Continuous epidural infusion of morphine for treatment of pain after thoracic surgery. Anesth Analg 63:757, 1984
43. El-Baz NM, Goldin M: Continuous epidural infusion of morphine for pain relief after cardiac operations. J Thorac Cardiovasc Surg 93:878, 1987
44. Allen PD, Walman T, Concepcion M et al: Epidural morphine provides postoperative pain relief in peripheral vascular and orthopedic surgical patients: A dose-response study. Anesth Analg 65:165, 1986
45. Gustafsson LL, Schildt B, Jacobsen KJ: Adverse effects of extradural and intrathecal opiates: Report of a nationwide survey in Sweden. Br J Anaesth 54:479, 1982
46. Chauvin M, Samii K, Schermann JM et al: Plasma morphine concentration after intrathecal administration of low doses of morphine. Br J Anaesth 53:1065, 1981
47. Bengtsson M, Lofstrom JB, Merits H: Postoperative pain relief with intrathecal morphine after major hip surgery. Reg Anesth 8:138, 1983
48. Katz J, Nelson W: Intrathecal morphine for postoperative pain relief. Reg Anesth 6:1, 1981
49. Chauvin M, Samii K, Schermann JM et al: Plasma pharmacokinetics of morphine after IM extradural and intrathecal administration. Br J Anaesth 54:843, 1981
50. Lazorthes Y, Gouarderes GH, Verdie JC et al: Analgesie par injection

intrathecale de morphine. Etude pharmacocinetique et application aux douleurs irreductibles. Neuro-Chirurgie 26:159, 1980

51. Nordberg G, Hedner T, Mellstrand T, Dahlström B: Pharmacokinetic aspects of intrathecal morphine analgesia. Anesthesiology 60:448, 1984

52. Abboud TK, Dror A, Mosaad P et al: Mini-dose intrathecal morphine for the relief of post-cesarean section pain: Safety, efficacy, and ventilatory responses to carbon dioxide. Anesth Analg 67:137, 1988

53. McQuay HJ, Sullivan AF, Smallman K, Dickenson AH: Intrathecal opioids, potency and lipophilicity. Pain 36:111, 1989

54. Hunt CO, Naulty JS, Bader AM et al: Perioperative analgesia with subarachnoid fentanyl-bupivacaine for cesarean delivery. Anesthesiology 71:535, 1989

55. Davies GK, Tolhurst-Cleaver CL, James TL: Respiratory depression after intrathecal narcotics. Anesthesia 35:1080, 1980

56. Gjessing J, Tomlin PJ: Postoperative pain control with intrathecal morphine. Anaesthesia 36:268, 1981

57. Jacobson L, Chabal C, Brody M: A dose-response study of intrathecal morphine: Efficacy, duration, optimal dose and side effects. Anesth Analg 67:1082, 1988

58. Johnson MD, Hurley RJ, Gilbertson LI, Datta S: Continuous microcatheter spinal anesthesia with subarachnoid meperidine for labor and delivery. Anesth Analg 70:658, 1990

59. Chadwick HS, Ready LB: Intrathecal and epidural morphine sulfate for post-cesarean analgesia—A clinical comparison. Anesthesiology 68:925, 1988

60. Bromage PK, Camporesi EM, Durant PA, Nielsen CH: Rostral spread of morphine. Anesthesiology 56:431, 1982

61. Bromage PR, Camporesi E, Leslie J: Epidural narcotics in volunteers. Sensitivity to pain and to carbon dioxide. Pain 9:145, 1980

62. Bromage PR, Joyal AC, Brinney JC: Local anesthetic drugs. Penetration from the spinal extradural space into the neuraxis. Science 140:392, 1963

63. DiChiro G: Movement of cerebrospinal fluid in human beings. Nature 204:290, 1964

64. DiChiro G: Observations on the circulation of the cerebrospinal fluid. Acta Radiol [Diagn] (Stockh) 5:988, 1966

65. Glynn CJ, Mather LE, Cousins MJ et al: Spinal narcotics and respiratory depression. Lancet ii:356, 1979

66. Camporesi EM, Nielsen CH, Bromage PR et al: Ventilatory CO_2 sensitivity after intravenous and epidural morphine in volunteers. Anesth Analg 62:633, 1983

67. Ngai SH, Berkowitz BA, Yang JC et al: Pharmacokinetics of naloxone in rats and man: Basis for its potency and short duration of action. Anesthesiology 44:398, 1976

68. Rawal N, Schött U, Dahlström B et al: Influence of naloxone infusion on analgesia and respiratory depression following epidural morphine. Anesthesiology 64:194, 1986

69. Gueneron JP, Ecoffey CI, Carli P et al: Effects of naloxone infusion on analgesia and respiratory depression after epidural fentanyl. Anesth Analg 67:35, 1988

70. Bromage PR, Camporesi EM, Durant PA, Nielsen CH: Nonrespiratory side effects of epidural morphine. Anesth Analg 61:490, 1982

71. Brownridge P: Epidural and intrathecal opiates for postoperative pain relief. Anaesthesia 38:74, 1983
72. Donadoni R, Rolly G, Noorduin H, Vanden Bussche G: Epidural sufentanil for postoperative pain relief. Anaesthesia 40:634, 1985
73. Welchew EA: The optimum concentration for epidural fentanyl. Anaesthesia 38:1037, 1983
74. Ready LB, Loper KA, Nessly M, Wild L: Postoperative epidural morphine is safe on surgical wards. Anesthesiology 75:452, 1991
75. Kotelko DM, Rottman RL, Wright WC et al: Transdermal scopalamine decreases nausea and vomiting following cesarean section in patients receiving epidural morphine. Anesthesiology 71:675, 1989
76. Loper KA, Ready LB, Dorman BH: Prophylactic transdermal scopalamine patches reduce nausea in postoperative patients receiving epidural morphine. Anesth Analg 68:144, 1989
77. Lawhorn CD, McNitt JD, Fibuch EE et al: Epidural morphine with butorphanol for postoperative analgesia after cesarean delivery. Anesth Analg 72:53, 1991
78. Bowdle TA, Greichen SL, Bjurstrom RL, Schoene RB: Butorphanol improves CO_2 response and ventilation after fentanyl analgesia. Anesth Analg 66:517, 1987
79. Davies GG, From R: A blinded study using nalbuphine for prevention of pruritis induced by epidural fentanyl. Anesthesiology 69:763, 1988
80. Baxter AD, Samson B, Penning J et al: Prevention of epidural morphine-induced respiratory depression with intravenous nalbupine infusion in post-thoracotomy patients. Can J Anaesth 36:503, 1989
81. Bromage PR, Camporesi E, Chestnut D: Epidural narcotics for postoperative analgesia. Anesth Analg 59:473, 1980
82. Ballantyne JC, Loach AB, Carr DB: Itching after epidural and spinal opiates. Pain 33:149, 1988
83. Durant PA, Yaksh TL: Drug effects on urinary bladder tone during spinal morphine-induced inhibition of the micturition reflex in unanesthetized rats. Anesthesiology 68:325, 1988
84. Thorén T, Tanghöj H, Mattwil M, Järnerot G: Epidural morphine delays gastric emptying and small intestinal transit in volunteers. Acta Anesth Scand 33:174, 1989
85. England DW, Davis IJ, Timmins AE et al: Gastric emptying: A study to compare the effects of intrathecal morphine and i.m. papaveretum analgesia. Br J Anaesth 59:1403, 1987
86. Bardon T, Ruckebusch Y: Comparative effects of opiate agonists on proximal and distal colonic motility in dogs. Eur J Pharmacol 110:329, 1985
87. Porreca F, Mosberg HI, Hurst R et al: Roles of mu, delta and kappa opioid receptors in spinal and supraspinal mediation of gastrointestinal transit effects and hotplate analgesia in the mouse. J Pharmacol Exp Ther 230:341, 1984
88. Gordh T Jr, Feuk U, Norlen K: Effect of epidural clonidine on spinal cord blood flow and regional and central hemodynamics in pigs. Anesth Analg 65:1312–1318, 1986
89. Eisenach J, Castro MI, Dewan DM, Rose JC: Epidural clonidine analgesia in obstetrics: Sheep studies. Anesthesiology 70:51–56, 1989
90. Rostaing S, Bonnet F, Levron JC, Vodinh J, Pluskwa F, Saada M: Effect

of epidural clonidine on analgesia and pharmacokinetics of epidural fentanyl in postoperative patient. Anesthesiology 75:420–425, 1991

91. Eisenach JC, Lysak SZ, Viscomi CM: Epidural clonidine analgesia following surgery: Phase I. Anesthesiology 71:640–646, 1989

92. Bonnet F, Bioco O, Rostaing S, Saada M, Loriferne JF, Touboul C, Abbay K, Ghignone M: Postoperative analgesia with epidural clonidine. Br J Anaesth 63:465–469, 1989

93. Bonnet F, Bioco O, Rostaing S, Loriferne JF, Saada M: Clonidine-induced analgesia in postoperative patients: Epidural vs. intramuscular administration. Anesthesiology 72:423–427, 1990

94. Gordh T Jr: Epidural clonidine for treatment of postoperative pain after thoracotomy. A double-blind placebo-controlled study. Acta Anaesthesiol Scand 32:702–709, 1988

95. Petit J, Oksenhendler G, Colas G, Leroy A, Winckler C: Comparison of the effects of morphine, clonidine and a combination of morphine and clonidine administered epidurally for postoperative analgesia (abstr). Anesthesiology 71:A647, 1989

96. Stenseth R, Sellevold O, Breivik H: Epidural morphine for postoperative pain: Experience with 1085 patients. Acta Anaesthesiol Scand 29:148–156, 1985

Pain Management in Cardiothoracic Surgery, edited by Gravlee and Rauck. J. B. Lippincott Company, Philadelphia © 1993.

Gale E. Thompson
Bernice R. Hecker

2 | Peripheral Nerve Blocks for Management of Thoracic Surgical Patients

With the exception of brachial plexus anesthesia, intercostal nerve block is the most useful peripheral nerve block. It is ideally suited for many applications in patients having cardiothoracic surgical procedures. Although it is one of the simplest and safest nerve blocks to perform, we believe that it remains one of the least utilized by the practicing anesthesiologist or intensivist. Misconceptions abound as to the safety of intercostal nerve block, especially with regard to the incidence of pneumothorax. Many seem to think that the time and effort necessary to perform the blocks pose formidable obstacles and that patient discomfort is great. These prejudices can be overcome by a proper understanding of the anatomy, physiology, and techniques of intercostal block.[1] The classic technique involves separate injections of each nerve in its individual intercostal space. This can be done in the midaxillary line or at any other more proximal site on the nerve including the paravertebral region. Is the risk and time investment of doing this block worth the "benefit" to be gained? The most significant future development to help answer this question would be the introduction of an ultralong acting (48–72 hours) local anesthetic drug to the marketplace. Having such a drug available would much more frequently direct this answer toward the benefit side.

Interpleural anesthesia represents a newer approach to intercostal nerve block that avoids some of the difficulties and hazards of multiple needle injections. First introduced in 1984, this technique is still evolving.[2] At present, its applications do not appear to be growing, but much more evaluation is necessary.[3] Continuous intercostal nerve block has been proposed as still another technique,[4] for which there is some supporting evidence. Critical evaluation would lead one to believe that this technique is often just interpleural anesthesia in disguise.

INTERCOSTAL NERVE BLOCK

Anatomy

The intercostal nerves are composed of the ventral rami of the 1st through 12th thoracic nerves.[5] The 1st, 2nd, and 12th differ from the other nine nerves in several respects. T_1 gives off a small contribution to the brachial plexus. T_2 and T_3 send cutaneous branches to the arm as the intercostobrachial nerve. T_{12} is not strictly an intercostal nerve, but rather a subcostal nerve that runs its course in the abdominal wall below the 12th rib and sends fibers to join the first lumbar nerve to help form the iliohypogastric and ilioinguinal nerves.

After exiting the vertebral foraminae, the intercostal nerves run a lateral course tucked into a groove on the underside of each rib. This groove is variable in manifestation and tends to diminish in depth and become a knife-like edge at around 12 to 15 cm from the vertebral spinous processes. Recent evidence from cadaver studies indicates that the classic medical school teaching of intercostal vein, artery, and nerve being located in precise order and comfortably tucked into the subcostal groove is somewhat unrealistic. The nerve may run a variable course from a subcostal to midcostal to supracostal location. Hardy found the frequency of these forms to be classical subcostal 16.6%, midzone 73%, and inferior supracostal 10% in his cadaver study.[6] Another anatomic subtlety for the anesthesiologist's appreciation concerns the matter of intercostal nerve branching which has two types. The nerve may split into separate bundles that have no common enclosing fascial sheath. These may rejoin or subdivide further as the nerve continues its lateral course, that is, there is not always a single well-defined nerve at every site in the intercostal space. Second, each intercostal nerve gives off four well-defined branches as it proceeds on its circuitous route anteriorly. The *first* is the gray rami communicans, which passes anterior to the sympathetic ganglion. The *second* branch arises as the posterior cutaneous branch and supplies skin and muscles in the paravertebral region. The *third* branch is the lateral cutaneous division, which arises just anterior to the midaxillary line. This branch is of primary concern when blocking the intercostal nerves for pain relief because it sends subcutaneous fibers coursing both posteriorly and anteriorly to supply skin of the chest and abdominal wall. The *terminal* or final branch is the anterior cutaneous branch, which provides cutaneous innervation to the midline of chest and abdomen. Unlike the situation posteriorly at the vertebral spines, there appears to be some slight overlap of sensory fibers across the midline of the chest and abdomen.

The paravertebral space deserves separate discussion. The dura mater and the arachnoid membrane fuse with the epineurium as the nerve exits the vertebral foramen. This has two important implications. Local anesthetic drugs (or other drugs) injected directly intraneurally may spread centrad to the nerve roots or spinal cord and produce anesthesia directly or indirectly by diffusing into the subarachnoid space. It is also possible to produce epidural anesthesia if a large volume of local anesthetic is injected into the paravertebral region and then flows centrad around the nerve in the vertebral foramen. Conocher has nicely demonstrated that even quick setting resin can be thus propelled into the vertebral epidural space.[7] He also showed that correctly placed paravertebral intercostal injections can readily spread over several intercostal spaces and even serve to dissect and reflect the pleura laterally from the vertebral bodies. In transverse section, the paravertebral space is wedge-shaped.[8] The posterior wall is the costotransverse ligament; anterolaterally is the parietal pleura; and medially lies the body of the vertebra and vertebral foramen. From the paravertebral space to the posterior angle of the rib, the intercostal nerve has no structure between it and the pleura. At the angle of the rib, the internal intercostal muscle arises and lies internal to the nerve all the way around to the costosternal cartilages.

In the paravertebral region the intercostal artery and vein are usually singular structures. Laterally they show multiple branches, which has implications for intercostal block because vessel puncture can lead to hematoma formation and/or rapid uptake of local anesthetic drug. Flank hematomas can become quite extensive in the anticoagulated patient. Other high risk scenarios include patients with neurofibromatosis, Marfan's syndrome, or arterial dilatation or stretching, for example, coarctation of the aorta or severe scoliosis.[9]

Technique

The Classic Approach

In the classic approach, intercostal nerve block is performed posteriorly at the angle of the ribs and just lateral to the sacrospinalis group of muscles. At this point the thickness of the rib is about 8 mm. Thus, if the needle is advanced 3 mm into the triangular fat-filled space wherein the nerve runs, there is a 5 mm margin of safety before penetrating the pleura. In most instances, the blocks are easiest to perform with the patient in a prone position with a pillow or roll placed under the midabdomen. This promotes optimum identification by palpation of the intercostal spaces posteriorly. The arms should be hanging over the sides of the table in order to rotate the scapuli laterally and make it easier to block the nerves of the upper ribs. After positioning the patient, it is helpful to use a skin-marking pen to identify the inferior edge of each rib. This serves as a map to illustrate and review anatomic detail and makes the process of blocking smoother and quicker. First, a vertical line is drawn down the posterior thoracic vertebral spines. Then, by palpation, the lateral edge of the sacrospinalis group of muscles is identified and marked as another vertical line. This line is usually about 7 to 8 cm from the posterior midline and has a tendency to angle medially at the upper levels. The inferior border of each rib is then marked along these two lateral vertical lines. (See Fig. 2–1)

Once these markings and local anesthetic mixing preparations have been completed, the initial step is to raise skin wheals (30 gauge needle) at each of the previously marked intersections of vertical and horizontal lines. A 2 to 3 cm, 22 or 23 gauge short bevel needle is then used to inject each intercostal nerve. If a disposable long-bevel needle is used, one must be aware that the tip may be easily bent with the repeated bony contacts required in doing this block. The needle can thus become barbed and potentially increase the risk for bleeding or nerve damage.

Hand and finger position is of utmost importance in performing this nerve block. (Fig. 2–2) Beginning at the lowest rib, a right-handed individual uses the index finger of the left hand to pull the skin at the lower edge of the rib cephalad and over the rib. The needle is then introduced to the rib as the anesthesiologist holds the syringe in the right hand. Should there be difficulty in contacting the rib, the palpating left index finger is used to redefine its depth and position. Obviously, care should be taken not to allow the needle to penetrate

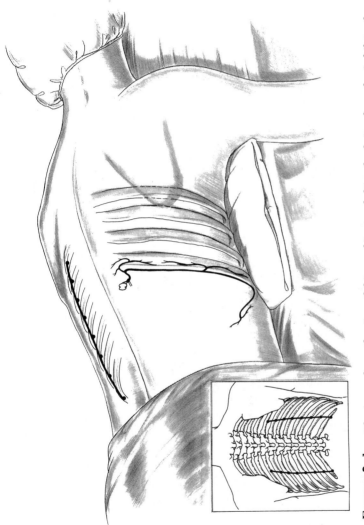

FIGURE 2–1.   The insert shows the sites of skin markings and skin wheal sites for a classic bilateral intercostal block. The figure illustrates patient position and a cross-sectional view through T_9 with the 4 branches of the nerve.

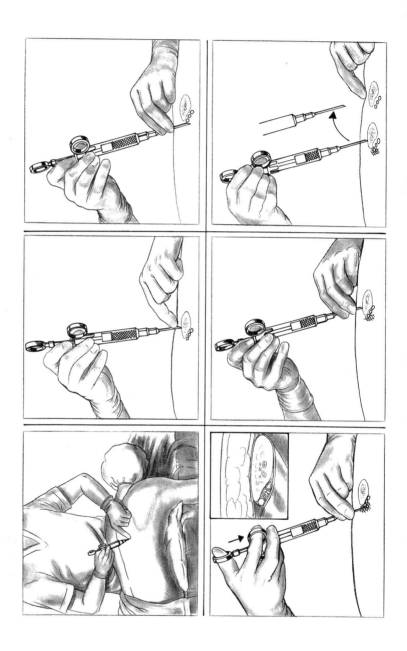

beyond this palpated depth because it could enter the interpleural or intra-alveolar space. While the right hand pushes to maintain firm contact between needle and rib, the left hand is shifted to gain control of the needle by holding the hub and shaft between thumb, index, and middle fingers. Firm placement of the left hypothenar eminence against the patient's back is crucial. This allows precise and constant control of needle depth as the left hand now "walks" the needle off the lower edge of the rib. If very slight pressure is applied to the plunger of the syringe by the right hand while the needle is being advanced, a loss of resistance is often felt as the needle enters this space. If properly done, the needle should be angled slightly cephalad. The needle is then grasped with the left hand, and 3 to 4 ml of solution is injected while gently moving the needle both inward and outward to initiate against the potential effects of intravascular injection. The left hand then walks the needle back onto the rib, and then releases the needle to free the index finger for palpation of the next higher rib. Keeping the needle on the previously injected rib serves to identify depth and avoid missing a rib or doing a repeat block of the same rib. The entire process is then repeated for each of the nerves to be blocked. An experienced individual can perform the entire procedure and successfully block 14 ribs in less than 5 minutes.

Midaxillary Approach

It is quite reasonable to perform intercostal nerve blocks in the midaxillary line. Some authors have advised against this process out of fear that it might be more prone to cause pneumothorax and to miss anesthetizing the lateral cutaneous branch of the nerve. Recall that this branch takes off near the midaxillary line and becomes superficial

---

FIGURE 2–2.   Intercostal nerve block; key steps in technique. (1) The right handed anesthetist stands to the left side of the prone patient. (2) After the skin is retracted over the rib, the needle is inserted to make firm contact with the rib. (3) The left hand is shifted to hold the needle and hub between the thumb and first two fingers before it is "walked off" the rib. The hypothenar eminence of the left hand always maintains firm contact with the patient's back. (4) The right hand is then shifted to occupy the three rings of the syringe; 3–5 ml solution is injected after the controlling left hand has inserted the needle tip 3–5 mm deeper than the caudad edge of the rib. (5) The right hand is shifted again and the left hand replaces the needle tip back onto the rib. (6) While the right hand maintains this position, the left index finger palpates the next higher rib and the entire sequence is repeated.

to innervate the skin of the anterolateral chest wall. However, two realities make intercostal block effective when done at a midaxillary site. First, the solution will always spread longitudinally in the intercostal groove for a distance of several centimeters from the site of injection. Second, one can inject the final milliliter of solution as the needle is being moved away from the rib toward the skin, which will anesthetize the lateral cutaneous branch in its subcutaneous location. Anesthesia of the abdominal wall results as does some degree of muscle relaxation, albeit less complete than when the block is done posteriorly. This approach makes intercostal block much more feasible in patients who cannot be turned supine or lateral, for example, the postoperative or trauma patient who experiences severe pain with any motion. This block can also be used to complement a general anesthetic technique after induction and intubation of a supine patient. The anesthesiologist can reach down and quickly do a series of unilateral or bilateral midaxillary or posterior axillary line blocks without even leaving the position at the head of the operating table. If the patient is being ventilated by an automatic ventilator during this time, it is advisable to synchronize the block with respiration rate, that is, avoid walking the needle off the rib at the point of maximum inspiration. This could help avoid pneumothorax.

The highest intercostal nerves can often be blocked by raising the patient's arm and palpating the ribs in the high axilla. One may also obtain good analgesia by blocking the intercostal nerve at even more anterior locations than the midaxillary line. For instance parasternal blocks can provide good pain relief after median sternotomy or fractures of the manubrium. Rectus sheath block is yet another variation.[5]

Paravertebral Approach

Intercostal blocks can be performed posteriorly at any site medial to the angle of the ribs. Obviously, there is some point at which a truly intercostal block becomes characterized as a paravertebral block. In some sense, the delineation is moot, but there are two very interesting observations: One is that central neuraxis spread of solution generates increasing concern as one moves medially, and that subpleural spread from one intercostal space to another also becomes more likely as one injects closer to the midline. Although Atkinson has stated that "paravertebral somatic block is now of more interest to historians than to practical anaesthetists," there are still reasons to explore this technique.[10] One is that catheters can be inserted here for a variation on the theme of interpleural anesthesia versus continuous intercostal nerve blockade. Truly the catheter would be extrapleural but similar efficacy and redosing principles apply.

It is immediately obvious that an errant thoracic paravertebral somatic or sympathetic nerve block might have significant physiological consequences because of the close proximity to vital structures. Central neuraxis spread of solution may result in subarachnoid or epidural anesthesia. Direct intravascular injection is always a possibility. Clearly, pneumothorax is also a significant risk. To perform this block, a skin wheal is raised 4 cm from the midline at the inferior edge of the rib to be blocked. It may be difficult to palpate the rib at this point because it angles steeply inward to its vertebral body attachments. However, if palpation is commenced laterally at the angle of the rib, it is usually possible to feel progressively more medial and thus define the rib, or to form a mental image of its origins. A 10 cm, 22 gauge needle is inserted perpendicular to the skin at the site of the skin wheal. Contact with the rib is usually made at a depth of 4 to 6 cm. With that depth now defined, the needle is withdrawn to a subcutaneous position and angled slightly medially and inferiorly before reinsertion. As it passes 1/2 to 1 cm deep to the rib, a total of 1 to 3 ml of local anesthetic solution is injected.

If a paravertebral catheter is to be used, the above described steps can be done using an 18 gauge Touhy needle to locate the loose areolar tissue of the paravertebral space deep to the rib. A catheter should be advanced only 1 to 2 cm beyond the tip of the needle as it could possibly enter the epidural space. A 3 ml test dose of local anesthetic drug should be used to detect intravascular or central neuraxis injection. Two or more catheters can be used for more extensive thoracoabdominal coverage as extrapleural spread of large volumes of local anesthetic can be unpredictable and increase the risk of epidural spread. Eason reports that one 15 ml injection can be expected to cover four intercostal spaces.[8]

Percutaneous Block via Jet Injection

A jet injection system has been designed and used for mass inoculations. This device has also been adapted to perform intercostal and other superficial peripheral nerve blocks without the use of needles. The injector jet is applied directly to the skin, but does not penetrate the skin. The injectate then passes topically on intraderinally to be subsequently absorbed into the blood stream. Other advantages include little or no risk of pneumothorax and rapid easy ability to perform multiple blocks. However, the procedure is not totally painless, transdermal spread of local anesthetic drug is unpredictable, and the jet gun has some major deficits. One is that only 1 ml of solution can be ejected per "shot." Although this could conceivably be overcome by other design, a larger ejected volume would likely be more painful. Seddon reported using 1 ml of 1.5% bupivacaine, which was specially prepared for the study as this concentration is not available commercially.[11] This drug concentration did not appear to be neurotoxic and the injection compared favorably with postoperative pain relief obtained by intramuscular narcotics in patients having cholecystectomy. Katz compared two separate 1 ml injections of 0.75% bupivacaine with a group of patients who received more traditional intercostal nerve blocks (3 ml) by needle injection.[12] It is interesting to note that neither group appeared to receive effective analgesia in that study.

Drug Dosages and Considerations

Sedative Drugs

All peripheral nerve block procedures for thoracic and abdominal analgesia utilize bony or vascular anatomic landmarks, and hence require no patient participation for proper execution of the block. Likewise, performance of these blocks may elicit significant skin and periosteal stimulation that can be obtained easily by light sleep or sedation. This is not to say that these nerve blocks cannot be performed without sedation. In fact, it may be mandatory to use minimal or no sedation when the blocks are performed on seriously ill patients. Drugs commonly used to supplement these blocks include midazolam, diazepam, fentanyl, ketamine, and the barbiturates. A wide variety of other drugs may also be used. The clinical situation dictates which one or ones should be used, depending on the need for hypnosis, analgesia, tranquilization, or some combination of effects. It is important to titrate them in small intravenous doses while observing closely for the desired action.

Local Anesthetic Drugs

As noted earlier, a desirable pharmacologic achievement for the near future would be the development of a local anesthetic agent with a predictable duration of action of 48 to 72 hours. There are problems in developing such a drug; chief among them being concerns about cardiac depression and neurotoxicity. At present there are short-acting (e.g., procaine), intermediate-acting (e.g., lidocaine), and long-acting (e.g., bupivacaine) local anesthetic drugs (Table 2–1). Before starting any regional anesthetic, the purpose or goal of the block must be determined by asking questions such as the following: "Do I want profound motor block, or is sensory anesthesia adequate?" "How many nerves are to be blocked?" "Is the patient going to be further anesthetized following the block, or will no supplementary drugs be given?" "Does the patient have major cardiovascular, respiratory, hepatic, or renal disease?" "What is the patient's size, body build, and age?" "Are there any special demands of this surgeon or of the surgical procedure?" Only when such questions have been answered can the anesthesiologist determine the proper volume, concentration, and dosage of local anesthetic drug. For instance, in preparing a solution of local anesthetic for bilateral intercostal nerve block, the following calculations are made:

Total volume of solution
Effective concentration of drug
Total (mg) dosage of drug
Volume of epinephrine to be added
Total dosage (μg) of epinephrine (Table 2–2)

There are safe or ideal limits for each of these interrelating factors. Volume multiplied by concentration determines total dose. Excesses of volume or concentration may be tolerated by some patients, but toxic effects are more likely to occur. On the other hand, small volumes or low concentrations of drug will result in ineffective regional anesthesia. Any block might be inadequate in area, duration, or degree of motor or sensory fiber blockade. The drug should be *tailored* to the block, which requires more than a vague knowledge of local

TABLE 2–1.   Drugs for Intercostal Block

Drug	Volume (ml)	Duration	Concentration	Dosage (mg/kg) Plain	Dosage (mg/kg) With Epi
Bupivacaine	60	8–12	0.5	2–3	2–3
Bupivacaine	60–100	6–12	0.25	2–3	2–3
Etidocaine	60–80	6–8	0.5	2–3	2–3
Tetracaine	60–100	5–9	0.10–0.15	2.0	2.0
Mepivacaine	60	4–8	0.5–1.0	7.0	9.0

TABLE 2–2.   Final Concentration of Epinephrine Derived From Total Dose and the Volume With Which It is Mixed

Epinephrine	Total Volume of Dilution	Final Concentration
0.1 mg in	20 ml =	1:200,000
0.2 mg in	40 ml =	1:200,000
0.25 mg in	50 ml =	1:200,000
0.25 mg in	60 ml =	1:240,000
0.25 mg in	80 ml =	1:320,000
0.25 mg in	100 ml =	1:400,000

anesthetic drug dosages and effective concentrations. The effective concentration will primarily depend on the drug used and the desired degree of motor nerve blockade. Table 2–1 shows some commonly used drugs and concentrations along with the range of acceptable volumes used for blocking intercostal nerves.

For each local anesthetic there are approved recommendations for maximum total dose. These recommendations may vary from country to country or region to region according to the prevailing bias or custom. Many regional techniques (e.g., subarachnoid block) require drug dosages that are far below the maximum recommended dose. However, to perform multiple bilateral intercostal blocks, the anesthesiologist will often need to approach the maximum recommended dose to achieve a successful block. Blood levels of a local anesthetic drug are higher after intercostal nerve bock than after any other of the commonly used regional anesthetic procedures. Tucker measured arterial plasma levels after epidural, caudal, intercostal, brachial plexus, and sciatic–femoral nerve block with a single injection of 500 mg of mepivacaine.[13] These blocks were performed with both 1% and 2% mepivacaine, with and without epinephrine. The highest plasma concentrations (5–10 μg/ml) were observed after intercostal nerve blocks without epinephrine. When a 1:200,000 concentration of epinephrine was added to the injected solution, plasma levels fell to the range of 2 to 5 μg/ml. These lower blood levels were similar to those found with all the other regional procedures measured. We prefer to add epinephrine to local anesthetic solution, both to reduce systemic absorption of local anesthetics and to potentially offset the myocardial depressant effects of bupivacaine. The presence of epinephrine also extends block duration for the shorter-acting local anesthetics.

Respiratory Effects

Intercostal blockade (ICB) produces effective analgesia with no central respiratory depression and minimal interference with pulmonary function. With the exception of peak expiratory flow (PEF), indices of respiratory function are essentially unaltered following ICB in healthy volunteers. Following thoracotomy, lung function is better in patients with ICB than in nonblocked controls.[14–18] Information from patients with underlying pulmonary disease is not available. However, our clinical experience indicates that ICB may be safely and effectively employed in patients with chronic obstructive pulmonary disease (COPD). Intercostal nerve blockade achieves excellent pain relief after thoracotomy in most patients.

Central Respiratory Control

Central respiratory drive is unimpaired following intercostal or cervicothoracic epidural blockade in healthy volunteers and patients.[19–21] The modified rebreathing test of Read examines the neuromuscular integrity of central respiratory drive. By comparing the response of minute ventilation (or other respiratory parameter) to a progressive rise in end-tidal CO_2 ($PETCO_2$), Read established this normally linear relationship as the "hypercapnic ventilatory response" (HCVR).[22] The slope of the line reflects the rate of change in ventilation (or other respiratory parameter) stimulated by increasing hypercapnia, and measures the sensitivity of the central respiratory center to changes in CO_2. The pCO_2 (or x) intercept of the line represents the "threshold" level of CO_2 below which the patient becomes apneic. Hypercapnic ventilatory response differs from individual to individual but is relatively constant for any one individual. Intercostal blockade changes neither the slope nor the x-intercept of the HCVR from control values.[19–21] This means that central ventilatory depression does not occur after ICB. Ventilation increases at the same level of stimulation and in the same magnitude as in unblocked controls. The pressure generated at the mouth during the first 100 msec of inspiration, $P_{0.1}$, is another test of central respiratory responsiveness.[23] Like the response of ventilation to hypercapnia, $P_{0.1}$ normally increases with hypercapnia. A change in $P_{0.1}$ with progressive hypercarbia occurs either when neural output or the efficiency of neuromuscular coupling (pressure attained for a given amount of muscle stimulation) changes. Hence, $P_{0.1}$ also reflects the impact of alterations in the mechanics of breathing on the respiratory system. Slopes and x-intercepts are the same for $P_{0.1}$ before and after ICB.[19] This means that ICB induces no central perception of neuromuscular dysfunction and does not interfere with the neurologic or muscular response of the respiratory system. After ICB in both seated and supine positions, the respiratory system responds appropriately and effectively. The increase in ventilation that normally occurs in response to hypoxia is also unaffected by ICB per se. However, in the immediate postoperative period, the presence of residual anesthetic agents obtunds the response to hypoxia. In this setting, assurance of adequate oxygenation requires oxygen saturation or arterial pO_2 monitoring regardless of the type of postoperative analgesia employed. Studies of ventilatory response in patients with COPD and ICB are not available. However, in healthy individuals, the effect on HCVR of expiratory viscous loading (airflow resistance) is established. Hecker and Schoene[19] reported unimpaired hypercapnic ventilatory responses in volunteers subjected to expiratory resistances of 6.5 cm H_2O with or without ICB. The combination of ICB and mild to moderate outflow resistance does not hamper the neuromuscular response to CO_2 stimulation.

Pulmonary (Lung) Function

Inspiratory Capacity

Although 20% to 30% of the inspiratory capacity normally depends on the external intercostal muscles, ICB does not interfere with seated or supine inspiratory capacity. In healthy, supine volunteers, ICB has no clinical effect on forced vital capacity (FVC), negative inspiratory effort (IE), maximum voluntary ventilation (MVV) or the inspiratory portions of maximal and partial flow-volume loops (inspiratory flow).[19] The stability of inspiratory capacity, from control through the establishment of high thoracic spinal and epidural blockade, confirms the findings reported with ICB.[24-26]

Postoperatively, two factors, pain and muscle spasm, are primarily responsible for the detrimental effects of thoracic or upper abdominal surgery on inspiratory capacity.[14,27] Pain directly inhibits deep breathing. By contrast, the analgesia associated with ICB facilitates inspiration. In addition, ICB prevents abdominal muscle spasm seen after thoracic or upper abdominal surgery. Duggan and Drummond[27] measured postoperative increases in the activity of the lower chest wall musculature (abdominals and lower intercostals). This activity is counterproductive. Muscle spasm mechanically impedes inspiration by increasing intra-abdominal pressure, which decreases respiratory system compliance, thus increasing the workload of the respiratory muscles. In addition, elevations in intra-abdominal pressure displace the diaphragm cephalad, which impairs diaphragmatic function by inhibiting the development of optimal diaphragmatic fiber length.[28,29] Intercostal nerve block eliminates or substantially reduces muscle tone. Postoperative patients with ICB inspire more deeply because of the ablation of pain and abnormal muscle activity. Vital capacity, an excellent indicator of inspiratory as well as expiratory capacity, is greater postoperatively in patients with ICB than in unblocked patients.[14–16]

Expiratory Capacity

Intercostal or high thoracic epidural blockade preserves expiratory function in healthy volunteers.[19,26,30,31] A statistically significant decrease in FVC occurs after ICB but the decrement is insignificant clinically. Flow-volume loop analysis demonstrates only a similar clinically insignificant decrease in PEF. Intercostal blockade has no effect on forced expiratory volume in one second (FEV1) in healthy volunteers (Table 2–3).

The positive effects of ICB on expiratory capacity are especially beneficial in postoperative patients. Reductions in vital capacity and FEV1 correlate with the incidence of postsurgical respiratory complications.[32,33] Measurements of these parameters, VC and FEV1, as well

TABLE 2–3. The Effects of ICB or High Epidural Blockade on the Dynamic Indices of Pulmonary Function in Nonoperated Volunteers or Patients

	Control	Block	Reference Numbers
VC (l)	5.73	5.28[a]	30
	6.36	6/13[a]	31
	5.53	5.18[a]	19
	2.99	3.07	26
PEF (l/sec)	10.88	9.93[a]	30
	10.54	10.08[a]	31
	11.23	9.25[b]	19
FEV$_1$ (l)	4.40	4.29	19
	2.48	2.59	26

[a]p < 0.05 for control vs. block; VC = vital capacity; PEF = peak expiratory flow; FEV$_1$ = forced expiratory volume in one second; l = liters. With the exception of [b], statistically different values do not represent clinically significant differences.

as PEF, are higher in postoperative patients with ICB than in un-blocked controls receiving intravenous or intramuscular opioids.[14-18] The improvement in these ventilatory indices associated with ICB provides a further incentive to perform the block (Table 2–4).

Lung Volumes

Normal inspiratory and expiratory capacities and flow maintain normal lung volumes. In healthy volunteers, the constancy of expiratory reserve volume (ERV), residual volume (RV), and functional residual capacity (FRC) after intercostal blockade is consistent with normal pulmonary capacity and function.[19] Studies of epidural or spinal blockade (to the T_6 dermatomal level) demonstrated similar findings.[24-26]

Pulmonary capacity and flow are not normal in postoperative patients. Upper abdominal and thoracic surgery adversely affect ventilatory mechanics. Reductions in VC, inspiratory capacity, and FRC mimic restrictive disease.[34] As components of the FRC, ERV and occasionally RV also decrease. Lower chest wall muscle spasm (cf. inspiratory capacity) and the experience of pain on deep inspiration negatively impact VC and inspiratory capacity and encourage rapid, shallow breathing. This abnormal pattern of ventilation contributes

TABLE 2–4. The Effects of ICB on the Dynamic Indices of Pulmonary Function in Postoperative Patients

	Control	ICB	Reference Numbers
VC(l)	36	76	14
	55	60	15
	25	56	16
PEF(l/sec)	39	82	14
	50	60	15
	32	57	16
FEV(l)	32	76	14
	55	63	15
	30	60	16
	28	31	17

Figures represent percentage of normal (presurgical baseline) value for patients with and without ICB (Control). All comparisons were made 24 hours after surgery and are significantly different. Values of ICB are greater than Control: VC, PEF and FEV_1 are greater during ICB. VC = vital capacity; PEF = peak expiratory flow; FEV_1 = forced expiratory volume in one second; l = liters.

to the decline in FRC seen several hours postoperatively. FRC and ERV reflect pulmonary reserve. The reduction in FRC (or ERV) is the most important mechanical aberration that occurs after surgery, and the one that correlates best with hypoxemia.[34] At reduced FRC, small airway closure occurs earlier in expiration because the distending pressure is less. This closure is most prominent in gravity-dependent areas where perfusion is best. Hence, pain and abnormal breathing patterns exacerbate ventilation–perfusion mismatch. Atelectasis develops if airway closure persists. Retained secretions, alterations in respiratory pattern and early airway closure are the major contributors to the development of atelectasis. A decrease in ERV far exceeds the importance of the other factors and may be the only factor required for the development of atelectasis.[35] Unlike narcotic-induced intravenous or intramuscular analgesia, ICB does not alter respiratory pattern or ERV. Postoperatively, ICB improves inspiratory and expiratory capacities and flows and, consequently, partially restores FRC and ERV. Intercostal blockade, then, acts to diminish the development of ventilation–perfusion mismatch and atelectasis. Arterial blood gas data support this analysis (cf. gas exchange).

Gas Exchange

Intercostal nerve blockade produces no change in arterial blood gases in supine, healthy volunteers.[31] After upper abdominal or thoracic surgery, examination of arterial blood gas data demonstrates a salutary effect of ICB on respiratory function.[15,18] Analgesia and attenuation of muscle spasm independently improve oxygenation and ventilation after ICB. Upper abdominal or thoracic surgery induces lower chest wall muscle spasm. Spasm interacts with postoperative alterations in central respiratory control to impair gas exchange.[34] In this environment, muscle relaxation may improve ventilatory mechanics and promote effective gas exchange. Analgesia enables patients to sit and ambulate earlier than patients without effective pain relief. The assumption of the seated or upright posture further improves gas exchange.

Clearance of Secretions

Reductions in PEF theoretically interfere with effective coughing, removal of secretions, and gas exchange. In healthy volunteers, the decrements in PEF after ICB are clinically insignificant. Recruitment of the triangularis sterni muscles (costosternal muscles; formerly, transversus thoracis) probably prevents more significant impairment.

The triangularis sterni work in concert with the abdominal muscles to produce expiratory force. Triangularis sterni and abdominal muscle activation appear to be neurally coupled. When development of abdominal muscle tension is inhibited, as by ICB, the triangularis sterni alone acts to markedly increase pleural pressure.[36] The expulsive force required to cough is sufficient as ICB leaves these muscles untouched. Further, postoperative pain suppresses the thoracic component of expiration[18] and attenuates deep inspiration, a necessary precondition for air expulsion. By providing anesthesia, ICB facilitates deep breathing, attendant lung recoil, and coughing.

Work: Normal Demand

The work of ventilation is directly proportional to the square of the tidal volume (Vt^2) and inversely proportional to the compliance (C') of the system: $Work \sim Vt^2/C'$. ICB alters neither tidal volume nor compliance during usual levels of ventilation. Under these conditions, the workload of the respiratory system as a whole is unaffected by ICB.

At equal minute ventilations, transdiaphragmatic pressure (Pdi) is the same before and after ICB in supine individuals (Unpublished, Hecker and Schoene). Transdiaphragmatic pressure reflects tension development in the diaphragm. The stability of Pdi means that the diaphragm performs the same amount of work before and after ICB. Nonetheless, metabolic rate (oxygen consumption) is significantly lower with increasing ventilatory demand in exercising healthy subjects with ICB as compared to unblocked controls.[19] One interpretation of these findings is that ventilation is more efficient. An alternative explanation is that overall oxygen demand is less because ICB inhibits the low-level tonic activity of a large mass of oxygen consuming muscle. During the postoperative period, this inhibition may decrease the work and oxygen demand of other respiratory muscles as well because reductions in respiratory system compliance[27] (which increase work) are prevented.

Intercostal blockade may promote diaphragmatic efficiency by other mechanisms after surgery. During restful supine breathing, ventilation is primarily dependent on the diaphragm. In the supine position, the ability of the diaphragm to increase its output is independent of thoracoabdominal muscle activity. The diaphragm operates from its optimal (least energy consuming) length–tension position because of the upward pressure of the abdominal contents on the diaphragmatic dome. The constancy of the FRC in blocked volunteers implies the maintenance of this length–tension relationship.

In postoperative patients, the partial restoration of FRC following ICB improves diaphragmatic configuration and confers some functional advantage.

Expiration normally does not require muscle activity. For the most part, lung compliance and recoil affect expiration and oxygen consumption is minimal. The stability or improvement in lung volumes, especially FRC and VC, suggests that after ICB overall respiratory system compliance remains normal in volunteers and improves in postsurgical patients.

In summary, ICB per se does not place an additional load on the respiratory system during inspiration or expiration. The mechanical alterations in ventilation induced by ICB do not increase oxygen demand. Indeed, these alterations decrease the metabolic rate until the demand for ventilation is extreme, $>120 \ 1 \cdot min^{-1}$.[19]

Underlying Disease and ICB

Intercostal blockade may be hazardous in patients with borderline pulmonary function or large or multiple bullae. A pneumothorax during nerve injection represents a potentially lethal complication and, ordinarily, unjustifiable risk in this group of patients. In less severely debilitated patients, ICB accomplishes useful goals without additional respiratory compromise.

Ventilation in COPD is adversely affected both by out-flow obstruction and, possibly, diaphragmatic mechanical disadvantage. The downward displacement of the diaphragm seen in patients with COPD theoretically reduces the effectiveness of diaphragmatic contraction and increases inspiratory dependence on the chest wall musculature. In patients with COPD, Sharp et al. demonstrated an increase in rib cage muscle activity that is consistent with this hypothesis.[38] The parasternal intercostals, scalene, and triangularis sterni muscles are responsible for this activity.[36,37] Intercostal blockade does not interfere with the function of these muscle groups. If rib cage compensation determines ventilation, ICB should be safe in patients with COPD.

More recent research indicates that diaphragmatic inspiratory action is well-preserved in patients with moderate to severe COPD.[39] Indeed, Pdis are higher at the same lung volumes among patients with COPD than among controls. The authors conclude that diaphragmatic function "is better" in patients with COPD because of length adaptation and possibly training hypertrophy.[39] Given unimpeded diaphragmatic output and facilitated secretion clearance, ICB is an appropriate technique in many patients with COPD.

Complications

Pneumothorax

The most feared complication of intercostal nerve block is pneumo-thorax. Many physicians avoid this block completely because they feel that the risk of producing this complication is high. However, with proper attention to technique the risk of pneumothorax should be extremely low. Moore has reported an incidence of pneumothorax of only 0.082% in an analysis of 17,000 patients. The majority of these blocks were done by residents in training.[40,41] Other authors have reported incidences of pneumothorax closer to 1% to 2%. In these series, the lesion was generally silent, asymptomatic, and discovered only because follow-up chest radiographs were taken.

An asymptomatic pneumothorax that can be found only on chest radiograph is of little clinical consequence and requires no treatment. On the other hand, an index of suspicion should always be maintained, and if a patient becomes symptomatic with chest pain or respiratory distress, a radiograph should be ordered. Treatment by needle aspiration or just careful observation is usually all that is necessary. Reabsorption of a small pneumothorax can be aided by administration of oxygen. Placement of a thoracostomy tube should be performed only if there is continued ventilatory embarrassment or a steady increase in the size of the pneumothorax.[42,43]

To produce a pneumothorax from an intercostal injection, the needle must puncture not only the parietal pleura, but also the visceral pleura. This will allow air to leak from the lung into the pleural cavity and can potentially even lead to a tension pneumothorax. The most common technical error that leads to this complication is improper positioning of the hands during the performance of the block. *For maximum safety, the hand that is advancing and controlling the needle must always be resting firmly on the patient's back.* If the patient moves suddenly, the hand and needle will then move in corresponding fashion.

Systemic Toxicity

A second source of complications from intercostal blocks is that of toxic effects of absorbed local anesthetic drugs. This problem is most likely to occur when large amounts of concentrated drug are injected to provide complete motor and sensory block in the surgical patient. Systemic toxic reactions are less likely in patients having diagnostic blocks or blocks performed for postoperative pain relief because smaller volumes of more dilute local anesthetic solution are ordinarily used in these cases. Absorption or intravascular injection of supra-convulsive doses interferes with conduction through sodium channels and causes vasodilation and myocardial depression—inotropic, chronotropic, and dromotropic. The presence of hypoxia lowers the threshold of occurrence.

Vasoconstrictive drugs retard local anesthetic absorption. Serum levels of local anesthetic following ICB with epinephrine and phenylephrine are comparable to those seen after other forms of regional anesthesia. In the serum ranges usually encountered after ICB, local anesthetics either have no effect on the myocardium or exhibit a minimally positive inotropic effect.[44] Generally, blood vessels dilate at the site of local anesthetic injection, but tone increases in some beds. Overall, the impact of the local anesthetic on the vasculature is less than that on the heart. Thus, in the usual situation, local anesthetic administration per se results in immediate small increases in cardiac output and arterial pressure. However, if serum concentrations are high, local anesthetics depress myocardial contractility and heart rate. Severe bradycardia and heart block with or without vasodilation impede resuscitation. Additives, like epinephrine and phenylephrine, markedly influence the cardiovascular system and complicate the picture described. β-adrenergic stimulation predominates with epinephrine. Tachycardia and increased contractility occur in proportion to the rate of absorption of these drugs (Table 2–5). If local anesthetic blood concentration is high, epinephrine inhibits toxic reactions and maintains cardiovascular function. Local anesthetic and epinephrine additively elevate cardiac output, heart rate, blood pressure, and, most important, oxygen consumption. Adjustments in drug administration are required to avoid stimulation in some patients. The incidence of tachycardia, dysrhythmias, and hypertension is low in healthy patients if the total dose of epinephrine is less than or equal to 0.3 mg and no direct intravascular injection occurs. Catecholamine-sensitive, hypertensive and thyrotoxic patients as well as patients with ischemic or other cardiac disease require more cautious treatment. A 0.2 mg total dose of epinephrine represents the upper limit to be considered in these patients. Phenylephrine is an alternative to epinephrine. Substitution of this drug prevents β-stimulation. Finally, some anesthesiologists delete vasoconstrictors when using highly protein-bound drugs, bupivacaine and etidocaine.[45]

In our own experience with over 5,000 blocks using bupivacaine (up to 400 mg), we have had 4 toxic reactions (0.08%).[40] Three of these

TABLE 2–5. Direct Cardiovascular Effects of Drugs Used to Induce Intercostal Blockade

	C.O.	HR	BP
LA: HIGH	↓↓	↓↓	↓↓
: USUAL	↑	→	↑
EPI	↑↑	↑↑	↑↑
PHENYL	Variable	↓	↑↑

LA = local anesthetic, high and usual = serum levels; CO = cardiac output; HR = heart rate; BP = blood pressure. (Modified from: Cousins MJ, Scott DB. Clinical pharmacology of local anesthetic agents. In Cousins MJ, Bridenbaugh PO (eds). Neural Blockade, 1st ed, p. 105 Philadelphia, J.B. Lippincott Co., 1980)

patients developed seizures within 15 minutes of completion of the block. Each case was treated by ventilating the patient with 100% oxygen and by controlling the seizures with small amounts of sodium thiopental. One additional patient developed severe cardiac depression following an intercostal block with 0.5% bupivacaine. The patient was an elderly woman and, because of history of angina, no epinephrine was added to the local anesthetic solution. Following the block, she developed a profound bradycardia and then asystole. This was treated with manual chest compression and an epinephrine infusion, which immediately restored heart rhythm and blood pressure.

Hypotension

A third complication that can occur is isolated hypotension. Cases in which this has been reported have occurred when intrathoracic blocks were performed under direct vision by the surgeon. It appears that in each case a high epidural or total spinal block resulted, and this subsequently led to a rapid and profound fall in blood pressure.[46–48] This problem has not occurred in surgical patients in whom the blocks were done percutaneously in the traditional manner.

We have also seen hypotension develop on occasion when intercostal blocks were done to provide postoperative pain relief for patients in the intensive care unit. Although the etiology is unclear, it appears that this occurs in patients who are possibly hypovolemic and who are also vasoconstricted because of severe pain. We hypothesize that when analgesia is produced by the intercostal blocks, the vasoconstriction ceases and the patient becomes hypotensive. Successful treatment in these cases is to use the Trendelenburg position and prompt administration of intravenous fluids. Because of the potential for this problem, it is always important to monitor vital signs carefully for 15 to 30 minutes following the performance of intercostal blocks.

Indications and Summary

In the operating room, intercostal blocks can be the cornerstone of a true balanced anesthetic technique. However, only a few surgical procedures can be performed under intercostal block alone. These include minor procedures on the chest or abdominal wall. In general, some degree of supplemental anesthesia must be used to complement the block or to facilitate and allow endotracheal intubation. In the operating room most patients will require supplementation with some combination of oxygen, nitrous oxide, or a low concentration of volatile anesthetic agent.

Outside of the operating room, there is no method of pain relief more effective for fractured ribs than intercostal nerve block. Chest wall contusion, pleurisy, and pain from flail chest can also be relieved. The pain from median sternotomy, pericardial window, or fractured sternum can be well controlled by blocks done in the parasternal region. Blockade of two or three nerves is a simple way to prepare for insertion of thoracostomy tubes and can provide analgesia for percutaneous biliary drainage procedures. Herpes zoster pain may be treated in this way. Intercostal nerve block can also be helpful in the differential diagnosis of visceral versus abdominal wall pain. Finally, the most effective, most important, but least exploited use of this block is for control of postoperative pain of the chest or abdomen.[49]

INTERPLEURAL ANALGESIA

Introduction

The first description of interpleural anesthesia by Kvalheim and Reiestad in 1984 was truly an innovative and astounding presentation.[2] As anatomy is a science that somewhat defies new concepts, it is amazing that a totally new perspective on regional anesthesia could be introduced at this time in history. Nonetheless, these authors introduced a novel and daring perspective to the practitioner of regional anesthesia. Many surgeons, and indeed many anesthesiologists, reacted startlingly to this new technique because of the boldness of a maneuver that would intentionally invade the somewhat sacrosanct interpleural space. There were obvious complications that sprang to mind, such as pneumothorax, lung abscess, and empyema. After many years of practicing intercostal block with the ever present dread of penetrating the pleural space as an integral caution, this approach of directly invading the interpleural space was almost too much to imagine. However, the technique does seem to be gradually gaining in acceptance and understanding, and is undergoing its own evolution.

In reality, one wonders whether the technique of interpleural anesthesia sprang de novo or whether it was a refinement of earlier work on paravertebral thoracic block and continuous intercostal block. In 1979, Eason[8] published a paper reappraising paravertebral thoracic block. His dissections clearly demonstrated the large variability in the course of the intercostal nerve. In clinical application, he introduced the use of catheters that could be inserted into the thoracic paravertebral space and used for repeated injections. He found that injection of 15 ml of 0.375% bupivacaine would consistently block at least 4 intercostal nerves. This was due to the fact that the single injection spread caudad and cephalad in the loose areolar tissue of the paravertebral space. Eason made injections through his catheters at a frequency of about every 4 hours and was able to very nicely control certain cases of postoperative pain in this manner. In 1980, an article by Nunn and Slavin[4] proposed a new anatomical basis for intercostal nerve block. They studied cadavers and evaluated the posterior part of the rib cage by fixation, decalcification, sectioning, and staining. Their studies showed that the intercostalis intimus muscle was a relatively flimsy structure composed of many fascicles and was loosely adherent to the posterior surface of the rib. This loose attachment allowed the free passage of India ink injections to go both caudad and centrad and to cover multiple intercostal spaces from one point of injection. This paper served to ignite considerable interest in what later was termed "continuous intercostal block." In 1983, Murphy[50] introduced the idea of inserting a catheter in one intercostal space and then intermittently injecting a large volume (20 ml of local anesthetic solution) to produce diffuse analgesia. His clinical success with this technique was followed by another study in cadavers in which he inserted catheters bilaterally into separate intercostal spaces and studied the postmortem spread of 20 ml of India ink.[51] The most interesting finding of his study was not that the India ink spread over several intercostal spaces, but that the integrity of the parietal pleura was found to be broken in a significant number of these cadavers when the pleural cavity was exposed. In reality, I believe this was one of the earliest demonstrations of interpleural anesthesia. Baxter and Flynn[52] also published a study in which they inserted catheters in 70 patients having cardiothoracic or abdominal surgery. In general, they found that the technique of single injection produced quite satisfactory analgesia. However, again the reality was that in some of these patients, the pleura was opened unintentionally during cardiac surgery and it was observed that the catheter was protruding into the interpleural space. Hence, this also was an early introduction of the concept of interpleural anesthesia. Nonetheless Kvalheim and Reiestad[2] deserve credit for defining interpleural anesthesia as a specific maneuver and for taking the step to insert the catheter directly into the interpleural space without describing the technique under other guises.

Technique

The technique for placing an interpleural catheter has been described in several ways. The original technique was to use a well-moistened 10 or 20 ml glass syringe that contained 2 to 4 ml of air. This syringe was attached to a 16 or 17 gauge Touhy epidural needle and inserted over the superior edge of the rib. This system was advanced as a single unit by moving the needle and lightly supporting the syringe. On entering the pleural space, the plunger was drawn down by the negative interpleural pressure and a small amount of air entered the pleural space from the syringe. The syringe was quickly removed and a small catheter inserted through the needle for a distance of 10 to 15 cm. This was in essence a closed technique at nearly all points. Another approach used "loss of resistance" as in epidural anesthesia. This technique seemed to lead to an unusually high complication rate in a study by Gomez, et al.,[53] in 1988. Yet another approach is to simply "walk off" the superior edge of the rib in a manner similar to that used for "walking off" the inferior edge of the rib in the classical intercostal block technique. One can do this with a 17 or 18 gauge Touhy needle, placing the needle on the basis of "feel" as one penetrates 3 to 5 mm deeper than the point of bony contact with the superior edge of the rib. This can be done with a stiletted needle or with a needle that is attached to a small 3 cc glass syringe. Another variation of catheter placement is that of direct placement of the catheter by the surgeon at the time of thoracotomy. This precise placement of the catheter can result in analgesia with lower dosages of local anesthetic drug.

Distribution and Absorption of Local Anesthetics

The distribution of local anesthetics injected into the interpleural space needs further definition. Stromskag[54] reported findings on computerized tomography taken 20 minutes after the injection of 20 ml of bupivacaine mixed with 10 ml of radiopaque contrast material. He evaluated patients who were placed in the supine position or the lateral position and found no significant difference in the cephalad–caudad distribution of contrast media between these two groups. Clinical use has certainly demonstrated that the patient's position is a very important factor in pooling of local anesthetic solution. For shoulder pain or stellate ganglion block, patients should be placed in a steep Trendelenburg position for the 15- to 20-minute period following injection. Likewise, if one intends to produce anesthesia in the lower thoracic or upper lumbar vertebral levels, the patient should be put in an extreme head up position following injection of the solution. The spread of local anesthetic will also be affected by the volume of local anesthetic injected. Most dosage regimens recommend anywhere from 20 to 30 cc of 0.25% to 0.5% bupivacaine for this technique. The peak serum levels of local anesthetic drug are reached between 10 and 20 minutes using these volumes of injected solution. The maximum plasma concentration of bupivacaine varied from 0.62 μg/ml in a group receiving 0.25% bupivacaine (20 ml) up to 1.20 μg/ml in a group receiving 0.5% bupivacaine (20 ml). The median duration of analgesia following injection was 285 minutes with the 0.25% solution and 500 minutes (range of 180–1080 minutes) in a group of patients receiving 0.5% bupivacaine.[55] Although the time between top-up doses was initially reported to be in the range of 5 to 26 hours, experience indicates that shorter intervals are more realistic.

MacIlvaine[56] described a technique of interpleural anesthesia in which he used a continuous infusion of bupivacaine for postoperative pain control in children. His dosage rate varied between 0.1 and 0.5 ml/kg/hr of 0.25% bupivacaine with epinephrine 1:200,000. He documented excellent pain relief but also demonstrated that the blood levels of local anesthetic drug reached extremely high concentrations after several hours. These peaked at 7 to 8 μg/ml of plasma in certain children, a concentration well above that considered toxic. It is thus apparent that patients can tolerate higher blood levels of local anesthetic drug from chronic infusion than from acute elevations to the same drug level, possibly because there is greater binding of bupivacaine by alpha acid glycoprotein as time passes. It is also apparent that the addition of epinephrine to the injected local anesthetic solution will decrease mean peak plasma concentrations of bupivacaine. Kambam et al.[57] report peak plasma concentrations of 0.32 μg/ml for epinephrine-containing bupivacaine versus 1.28 μg/ml for nonepinephrine containing solutions with a similar volume (20 ml) injected into both groups of patients. There is little doubt about the efficacy of interpleural anesthesia in controlling postoperative pain in a variety of surgical patients.[56] The technique was initially used primarily for unilateral surgical incisions such as cholecystectomy, nephrectomy, and mastectomy. Other applications of the technique have been for the control of pain from multiple rib fractures and for diagnostic and therapeutic blocks in patients experiencing pain of pancreatic origin.[58,59] The injected local anesthetic drug reaches the mediastinal region and can produce block of the sympathetic chain as evidenced by observation of Horner's syndrome in some patients. The technique has also been used for treatment of postherpetic neuralgia.[60]

Complications and Side Effects

There are few complications of interpleural anesthesia reported thus far. Obviously, pneumothorax heads the list. This seems to be a rare event but it appears more likely when the pressure release technique of insertion of the catheter has been used and a long length (i.e., 30 cm) of catheter insertion follows. It is unclear as to when pneumothorax may manifest on x-ray study. Perhaps, by definition, there is a small pneumothorax in every patient as 10 to 20 ml of air might be sucked in during the catheter insertion. One tension pneumothorax has been reported.[63] Other complications include toxic systemic reactions to the local anesthetic drug and pleural effusion. Horner's syndrome and catheter rupture have also been seen. Complications of catheter placement include insertion of the catheter directly into the substance of the lung or into necrotic tumors. Infection has been reported in a small number of patients.[58,61] The obvious question is whether this was due to the catheter or secondary to surgery. Systemic toxic reactions have also occurred following local anesthetic injection. In one report, a patient developed toxic symptoms following 30 ml of 0.75% bupivacaine. The arterial serum concentration of bupivacaine was 6 μg/ml. In another report of systemic toxicity, 20 ml of 2% lidocaine was injected and the resultant serum concentration reached a peak of 4.7 μg/ml. The patient experienced muscle twitches, tachycardia, hypertension, and some sense of disorientation. Grand mal seizures were observed in one patient after injection of 30 ml of 0.5% bupivacaine. The measured serum concentration was 4.9 μg/ml.

CRYOANALGESIA

In 1976, Lloyd et al.[62] coined the term cryoanalgesia to describe a new method of achieving pain relief by using extreme cold for temporary disruption of nerve conduction. The concept of cold analgesia anesthesia is as cold as the history of man, but the technique described by Lloyd[62] introduced a new method of generating and applying the cold via a 15-gauge cryoneedle which could produce temperatures to around −75°C at its tip. This temperature was created by utilizing the Joule–Thompson effect, that is, a stream of compressed gas suddenly expands and cools. The hope for this technique was that it would produce a temporary kind of nerve destruction without the heavy scarring and neuroma formation that is likely to occur after other methods of neurolysis. Histologic studies supported this idea as there was minimal destruction of the endoneurium, and in animals normal nerve function returned after several weeks. Clinically the technique found greatest application for intercostal nerve block performed internally by the surgeon just before closing a thoracotomy.[63,64] Thus the nerve could be easily dissected free of its surrounding blood vessels and the cold applied specifically to the nerve. Although somewhat tedious, this process could be done by an appropriately enthusiastic surgeon and some studies showed a decrease in postoperative narcotic requirements in patients to whom this was done. However, narcotic use was never completely eliminated and one is left to wonder whether more nerves should have been blocked or if the temperature was properly applied for a long enough duration. Other cautions with the technique include the potential to damage surrounding tissue by withdrawing a still frozen probe and the potential for cold damage to the adjacent spinal cords or its arterial supply. The total extent or peripheral limits of the cold damage is difficult to accurately define, and the technique has never achieved widespread popularity.

References

1. Moore DC, Bridenbaugh LD: Intercostal nerve block in 4333 patients: Indications, technique, and complications. Anesth Analg 41:1, 1962
2. Kvalheim L, Reiestad F: Interpleural catheter in the management of postoperative pain. Anesthesiology 61:A231, 1984
3. Covino BG: Interpleural regional anesthesia. Anesth Analg 67:42, 1988
4. Nunn JF, Slavin G: Posterior intercostal nerve blocks for pain relief after cholecystectomy. Br J Anaesth 52:253, 1980
5. Thompson GE, Brown DL: The common nerve blocks. In Nunn JF, Utting JE, Brown BR (eds). General Anaesthesia, 5th ed., p. 1070. London, Butterworth, 1989
6. Hardy PAJ: Anatomical variation in the position of the proximal intercostal nerve. Br J Anaesth 61:338, 1988
7. Conacher ID: Resin injection of thoracic paravertebral spaces. Br J Anaesth 61:657, 1988
8. Eason MJ, Wyatt R: Paravertebral thoracic block—A reappraisal. Anaesthesia 34:638, 1979
9. Butchart EG, Grott GJ, Barnsley WC: Spontaneous rupture of an intercostal artery in a patient with neurofibromatosis and scoliosis. J Thorac Cardiovasc Surg 69:919, 1975
10. Atkinson RS, Rushman GB: A synopsis of anaesthesia, 8th ed., p. 387., Bristol, England, John Wright & Sons Ltd., 1977
11. Seddon SJ: Intercostal nerve block by jet injection. Anaesthesia 39:484, 1984
12. Katz J, Knarr D, Juneja M: Intercostal nerve block by jet injection. Anesthesia 75:A726, 1991
13. Tucker GT, Moore DC, Bridenbaugh PO: Systemic absorption of mepivacaine in commonly used regional block procedures (abstr). Anesthesiology 37:277, 1972
14. Mozell EJ, Sabanathan S, Mearns AJ, Bickford-Smith PJ, Majid MR, Zografor G: Continuous extrapleural intercostal nerve block after pleurectomy. Thorax 46:21, 1991
15. Engberg G: Respiratory performance after upper abdominal surgery. A comparison of pain relief with intercostal blocks and centrally acting analgesics. Acta Anesth Scand 29:427, 1985
16. Sabanathan S, Mearns AJ, Bickford-Smith PJ, Eng J, Berrisford, Bibby SR, Majid MR: Efficacy of continuous extrapleural intercostal nerve block on post-thoracotomy pain and pulmonary mechanics. Br J Surg 77:221, 1990
17. de la Rocha AG, Chambers K: Pain amelioration after thoracotomy: A prospective, randomized study. Ann Thorac Surg 37:239, 1984

18. Pedersen VM, Schulze S, Hoier-Madsen K, Halkier E: Air-flow meter assessment of the effect of intercostal nerve blockade on respiratory function in rib fractures. Acta Chir Scand 149:119, 1983

19. Hecker BR, Fjurstrom R, Schoene RB: Effect of intercostal nerve blockade on respiratory mechanics and CO_2 chemosensitivity at rest and exercise. Anesthesiology 70:13, 1989

20. Dohi S, Takeshima R, Naito H: Ventilatory and circulatory responses to carbon dioxide and high level sympathectomy induced by epidural blockade in awake humans. Anesth Analg 65:9, 1986

21. Sakura S, Saito Y, Maeda M, Kosaka Y: Epidural analgesia in Eaton–Lambert myasthenic syndrome. Anaesthesia 46:560, 1991

22. Read DJ: A clinical method for assessing the ventilatory response to carbon dioxide. Aust Ann Med 16:20, 1976

23. Schoene RB, Pierson DJ, Butler J: Constancy of functional residual capacity in the supine position during hypoxia and hyperoxic hypercapnia. Am Rev Respir Dis 124:508, 1981

24. Freund FG, Bonica JJ, Ward RJ, Akamatsu TJ, Kennedy WF: Ventilatory reserve and level of motor block during high spinal and epidural anesthesia. Anesthesiology 28:834, 1967

25. Wahba WM, Craig DB, Don HF, Becklake MR: The cardio-respiratory effects of thoracic epidural anaesthesia. Can Anaesth Soc J 19:8, 1972

26. McCarthy GS: The effect of thoracic extradural analgesia on pulmonary gas distribution, functional residual capacity and airway closure. Br J Anaesth 48:243, 1976

27. Duggan J, Drummond GB: Activity of lower intercostal and abdominal muscle after upper abdominal surgery. Anesth Analg 66:852, 1987

28. Nunn JF: Applied Respiratory Physiology, 3rd ed., p. 89. London: Butterworths, 1987

29. Kim MJ, Druz WS, Danon J, Machnach W, Sharp JT: Mechanics of the canine diaphragm. J Appl Physiol 41:369, 1976

30. Jakobson S, Ivarsson I: Effects of intercostal nerve blocks (bupivacaine 0.25% and etidocaine 0.5%) on chest wall mechanics in healthy men. Acta Anesth Scand 21:489, 1977

31. Jakobson S, Fredriksson H, Hedenstrom H, Ivarsson I: Effects of intercostal nerve blocks on pulmonary mechanics in healthy men. Acta Anesth Scand 24:482, 1980

32. Meyers JR, Lembeck L, O'Kane H, Baue AE: Changes in functional residual capacity of the lung after operation. Arch Surg 110:576, 1975

33. Alexander JI, Spence AA, Parikh RK, Stuart B: The role of airway closure in postoperative hypoxaemia. Br J Anaesth 45:34, 1973

34. Craig DB: Postoperative recovery of pulmonary function. Anesth Analg 60:46, 1981

35. Tisi GM: Preoperative evaluation of pulmonary function. Am Rev Respir Dis 119:293, 1979

36. De Troyer A, Ninane V, Gilmartin JJ, Lemerre C, Estenne M: Triangularis sterni muscle use in supine humans. J Appl Physiol 62:919, 1987

37. De Troyer A, Estenne M: Coordination between rib cage muscles and diaphragm during quiet breathing in humans. J Appl Physiol 57:899, 1984

38. Sharp JT, Goldberg NG, Druz WS, Fishman HC, Danon J: Thoracoabdominal motion in chronic obstructive pulmonary disease. Am Rev Respir Dis 115:47, 1977

39. Similowski T, Yan S, Gauthier AP, Macklem PT, Bellemare F: Contractile properties of the human diaphragm during chronic hyperinflation. N Engl J Med 325:917, 1991

40. Moore DC, Bridenbaugh LD: Pneumothorax: Its incidence following intercostal nerve block. JAMA 182:1005, 1962

41. Moore DC: In Benedetti D (ed). Advances in Pain Research and Therapy. Intercostal nerve block and celiac plexus block for pain therapy. Volume 7:309. New York, Raven Press, 1984

42. Jones JS: A place for aspiration in the treatment of spontaneous pneumothorax. Thorax 40:66, 1985

43. Vallee P: Sequential treatment of a simple pneumothorax. Ann Emerg Med 17:936, 1988

44. Jorfeldt L et al: The effect of local anesthetics on the central circulation and respiration in man and dog. Acta Anesth Scand 12:153, 1968

45. Tucker GT, Mather LE: Pharmacokinetics of local anesthetic agents. Br J Anaesth 47:213, 1975

46. Benumof JL, Semenza I: Total spinal anesthesia following intrathoracic intercostal nerve blocks. Anesthesiology 43:124, 1975

47. Skretting P: Hypotension after intercostal nerve block during thoracotomy under general anesthesia. Br J Anaesth 53:527, 1981

48. Sury MRJ, Bingham RM: Accidental spinal anesthesia following intrathoracic intercostal nerve blockade. Anaesthesia 41:401, 1986

49. Bridenbaugh PO, DuPen SL, Moore DC et al: Postoperative intercostal nerve block analgesia versus narcotic analgesia. Anesth Analg 52:81, 1973

50. Murphy DF: Continuous intercostal nerve blockade for pain relief following cholecystectomy. Br J Anaesth 55:521, 1983

51. Murphy DF: Continuous intercostal nerve blockade: An anatomical study to elucidate its mode of action. Br J Anaesth 56:627, 1984

52. Baxter AD, Flynn JF, Jennings FO: Continuous intercostal nerve blockade. Br J Anaesth 56:665, 1984

53. Gomez MN, Symreng T, Johnson B, Rossi NP, Chiang CK: Intrapleural bupivacaine for intraoperative analgesia—A dangerous technique? Anesth Analg 67:S78, 1988

54. Stromskag KE, Hauge O, Steen PA: Distribution of local anesthetics injected into the interpleural space, studied by computerized tomography. Acta Anesth Scand 34:323, 1990

55. Stromskag KE, Reiestad F, Holmquist EVO, Ogenstad S: Intrapleural administration of 0.25%, 0.375% and 0.5% bupivacaine with epinephrine after cholecystectomy. Anesth Analg 67:430, 1980

56. McIlvaine WB, Knox RF, Fennesseyt PV, Goldstein M: Continuous infusion of bupivacaine via interpleural catheter for analgesia after thoracotomy in children. Anesthesiology 69:261, 1988

57. Kambam JR, Hammon J, Parris WCV, Lupinetti FM: Intrapleural analgesia for postthoracotomy pain and blood levels of bupivacaine following intrapleural injection. Can J Anaesth 36:106, 1989

58. Ahlburg P, Noreng M, Molgaard J, Egebo K: Treatment of pancreatic pain with interpleural bupivacaine: An open trial. Acta Anesth Scand 34:156, 1990

59. Reiestad F, McIlvaine WB, Kvalheim L, Haraldstad P, Pettersen B: Successful treatment of chronic pancreatic pain with interpleural analgesia. Can J Anaesth 36:713, 1989

60. Sihota MK, Holmblad BR: Horner's syndrome after interpleural anesthesia with bupivacaine for post-herpetic neuralgia. Acta Anesth Scand 32:593, 1988

61. Stromskag KE, Minor B, Steen PA: Side effects and complications related to interpleural analgesia: An update. Acta Anesth Scand 34:473, 1990

62. Lloyd JW, Barnard JDW, Glynn CJ: Cryoanalgesia, a new approach to pain relief. Lancet ii:932, 1976

63. Glynn CJ, Lloyd JW, Barnard JDW: Cryoanalgesia in the management of post-thoracotomy pain. Thorax 35:325, 1980

64. Maiwand O, Makey AR: Cryoanalgesia for relief of pain after thoracotomy. Br Med J 282:1749, 1981

Pain Management in Cardiothoracic Surgery, edited by Gravlee and Rauck. J. B. Lippincott Company, Philadelphia © 1993.

Richard L. Wolman

3 | Patient-Controlled Analgesia Following Thoracic Surgery

Numerous techniques are utilized for pain control following thoracic surgery. Patient-controlled analgesia (PCA) is one such method. This chapter develops this subject by first presenting the problems with inadequate postoperative analgesia and with nonpatient-controlled analgesic techniques, and then reviews the subject of patient-controlled analgesia. Whenever possible, emphasis has been placed on thoracic surgical applications of this technique, but the rather sparse literature on this specific PCA application mandates that much of the discussion not be specific for thoracic surgical patients. Much of the theory and extensive PCA practice derived from other surgical incision sites should transfer to thoracic surgery, but more studies comparing PCA to other analgesic techniques in thoracic surgical patients are needed. It is hoped that this discussion will prompt some readers to perform these studies.

THE PROBLEM OF INADEQUATE POSTOPERATIVE ANALGESIA

Despite sophisticated technological advances in all disciplines of medicine, we have, as a profession largely failed to provide relief from acute postoperative pain.[1-12] Nowhere is this problem more evident than after thoracic surgery. The problem of pain is not new to our generation of physicians as the quest for analgesia dates back some 62,000 years to Neanderthal times.[13] According to the *British Medical Journal*, "it is an indictment of modern medicine that such a simple problem as the relief of postoperative pain remains largely unsolved."[14] The problem of postoperative pain management is not simple. Attempts to find an individual patient's analgesic window are complicated by both interpatient and intrapatient variability in analgesic requirements.[15] Nowhere is this more of a problem than after thoracic surgery, where pain is severe.[16]

The scope of inadequate postoperative analgesia is enormous. There are approximately 53 million surgical procedures performed each year in the United States, and somewhere between 33% and 75% of patients complain of moderate to severe postoperative pain despite treatment.[3,4,5,6,7,17,18] In addition, of 75 million patients suffering traumatic injuries per year in the United States, over one third complain of moderate to severe pain.[19]

What is pain? Pain is an unpleasant sensory and emotional experience associated with actual or potential tissue damage or described in terms of such damage.[20] Therefore, pain is not simply a sensation. Rather, it is a complex subjective perception of a noxious stimulus, real or imagined.[20–22] As it is a subjective phenomenon, pain is difficult to quantify,[23] and, therefore difficult for those trained in concrete analysis to appreciate. Pain has three components: sensory, evaluative, and affective.[24] As such, it may be described by magnitude, quality, and psychological components.

Acute pain has been defined as "a complex constellation of unpleasant sensory, perceptual and emotional experiences and certain associated autonomic, psychologic, emotional, and behavioral responses"[25] provoked by injury, acute disease, or tissue dysfunction with or without tissue damage. It is usually biologically useful, warning the patient that something is wrong and evoking stillness, which promotes healing. The neuroendocrine stress response that it provokes may help the individual deal with the disease or injury. Acute postoperative pain, a variant of acute pain, is usually not biologically useful, and the resultant stress response is usually harmful to the patient.

There are two components of acute pain—background and acute response pain.[26] Background pain is what the patient experiences while at rest. Acute response pain is what the patient experiences during activities such as manipulations, cough, deep breathing, dressing changes, mobilization, physical therapy, and the like. As such, acute response pain is transient. Each component of acute pain must be effectively treated without over- or underdosing the patient and each component should decrease as the patient recovers.

CONSEQUENCES OF INADEQUATE POSTOPERATIVE ANALGESIA

Humanitarian reasons alone dictate the need to control acute pain. However, acute pain also needs to be controlled because it increases patient morbidity, mortality, and medical costs to the patient and society as a whole. Acute pain results in an increase in pulmonary, cardiovascular, coagulation, gastrointestinal, and psychological complications, and an increase in the neurohumoral stress response.

Nontreated or ineffectively treated acute pain causes a reversible restrictive pulmonary picture with decreases in vital capacity (50%–75%) and functional residual capacity (FRC). This results in a significantly greater ventilation–perfusion mismatch and alveolar–arterial oxygen tension difference than that seen in effectively treated patients.[27] The incidence of pulmonary complications increases when the postoperative FRC decreases to 60% of the preoperative value, with more severe complications occurring at 40%.[28] Splinting after thoracic or upper abdominal surgery results in atelectasis, failure to cough and clear secretions, mucus plugging of airways, pneumonia, hypoxia, and hypercarbia. Hence, acute pain may result in a decrease in tissue oxygen supply. Effective postoperative analgesia, especially following thoracic surgery, is mandatory to reverse this decrease in pulmonary function and is vital for an uncomplicated recovery.[29]

Acute pain also increases catecholamine release, sympathetic activity, and oxygen consumption and, therefore, a potential disequilibrium in myocardial oxygen supply and demand. Increased myocardial oxygen demand (e.g., hypertension, tachycardia) coupled with a decreased oxygen supply (e.g., hypoxemia, tachycardia) increases the risk of myocardial ischemia.

Inadequate analgesia necessitates immobilization, which may cause venous pooling. Coupled with increased platelet aggregation, this places the patient at risk for deep venous thrombosis and pulmonary emboli. Gastrointestinal side effects of pain, such as gastric stasis and ileus, further complicate treatment and recovery.

The neurohumoral stress response to surgery is similar to that following injury.[30] In addition to the response mediated by kinins, leukotrienes, and prostaglandins[31] there is increased release of cate-cholamines and secretion of adrenocorticotropic hormone (ACTH) and glucagon,[32,33] which results in hyperglycemia, insulin resistance, gluconeogenesis, lipolysis, and protein catabolism.[34,35] Although controversial, it appears that analgesia may blunt this stress response.[36-41]

Finally, inadequately managed acute pain may result in a pain–symptom complex with long-term chronic pain implications.[42] This cyclic complex of pain, anxiety, fear, hostility, loneliness, sleep deprivation, and helplessness may be the reason for the "intensive care syndrome"[43] or "ICU psychosis." At the very least the patient may become a psychological cripple, unable to cope with pain and stress or to participate in his or her own treatment. All of these side effects resulting from injury or inadequate analgesia may delay recovery, increase morbidity and mortality, and increase the cost of medical care to the patient and society as a whole.

WHY INADEQUATE POSTOPERATIVE ANALGESIA? WHO IS AT FAULT?

Given the advances in pharmacologic agents as well as other areas of medicine, it seems illogical that patients would still suffer from acute postoperative pain. Yet our lack of understanding of the individual nature of acute postoperative pain coupled with ignorance regarding analgesic agents, especially their potency and side effects, has resulted in a perhaps "abnormal concern" for side effects.[3,4] In fact, Angell editorialized in 1982 that "in no other area of medicine has such an extravagant concern for side effects so drastically limited treatment."[11]

Despite the evidence,[1-12] the problem of inadequate analgesia continues. Serious deficiencies in standard analgesic regimens were noted as early as 1956,[44] and by 1961 it was shown that routine regimens of postoperative analgesia were inadequate.[7] Marks and Sachar in 1973 and Donovan et al. in 1987 demonstrated that hospitalized patients were only receiving one quarter of their prescribed analgesics even though they were experiencing inadequate analgesia[5,45] and sleep disturbances.[45]

The blame for mismanagement of acute pain rests with physicians, nurses, and patients.[46] Physicians may be unwilling to use consulting services or embark on unfamiliar treatment protocols such as PCA, continuous infusion of intravenous narcotics, regional anesthetic techniques, or epidural or intrathecal narcotics. Orders for commonly used opioids may be inadequate based on agent, dose, dose interval, use of ranges of doses or time intervals, or use of prn administration. Nurses may use the lowest dose and longest time intervals between doses, or there may be a time delay between patient requests and administration of the agent. Finally, patients may be either unable or unwilling to communicate their analgesic needs (based on age, language, intelligence, ethnic, cultural or psychological background, fear, or physical impairment) or unwilling to consent to analgesic remedies different from their expectations due to fear of the unknown.

In an attempt to understand the basis for inadequate analgesia, Weis and colleagues surveyed housestaff and nurses regarding postoperative analgesic care.[4] Despite the fact that 41% of the patient population complained of moderate to severe postoperative pain, 54% of the M.D.s and 74% of the nurses thought that the patients received adequate analgesia. Only one fifth of the physicians prescribed for complete pain relief. These discrepancies were based on a lack of confidence in using opioid analgesics resulting from inadequate knowledge of pharmacology; misconceptions regarding drug combinations, addictive potential, and respiratory depression; and misconceptions regarding interpretation of the placebo response and fictitious pain. Other possible sources of error include ignorance of inter- and intrapatient variability and changes in the pharmacokinetics and pharmacodynamics of analgesic agents in this population. Mather and Phillips [46] have defined six misconceptions regarding opioid use in acute pain:

"1. Doses should be as small and infrequent as possible to avoid the development of addiction.
2. Doses larger than the standard do not increase pain relief and cause heavy sedation and respiratory depression.
3. Nursing and/or medical staff know when and how much pain relief each patient needs.
4. Patients requesting more pain relief than the standard are psychologically abnormal or are becoming addicted.
5. If non-opioid drugs are ordered, these should be tried in preference to opioids.
6. What is needed is a powerful nonaddictive pain reliever."

To these misconceptions add:

7. Immobile, paralyzed, intubated, and mechanically ventilated patients do not hurt.
8. Analgesia renders the critically ill patient hemodynamically unstable.

These misconceptions are based on greatly exaggerated fears regarding the analgesic potency of opioids and their effects on the patient: respiratory and circulatory integrity, addiction, physical dependence, and tolerance. Fears of addiction, tolerance, and dependence are not substantiated in the literature. Iatrogenic dependence is rare (less than 0.1%) in hospitalized patients experiencing acute pain[47,48] and tolerance is easily treated and rarely a clinical problem. Opioid induced respiratory depression is rare (0.9%) in postoperative patients[49] and even the critically ill can be made analgesic with the proper use of common opioids without respiratory or cardiovascular depression.[50]

THE IDEAL ANALGESIC AGENT

The ideal agent for producing analgesia in the postoperative patient would work at a specific receptor or subset of receptors to give a measured, desired result without side effects. It would be easy to administer; offer multiple possible routes of administration; have a rapid onset of action; be fully predictable in its effect, duration of action, metabolism, and excretion; cause minimal side effects; induce minimal tolerance; have little or no potential for psychological addiction or physical dependence; and be inexpensive and readily available. This ideal drug would by definition have a high therapeutic index.[51,52]

In spite of considerable research in the field of new drug development, no specific agent satisfies all of these criteria. It has been the physicians' responsibility to tailor an analgesic regimen to meet each individual patient's needs. We obviously have failed as inadequate postoperative analgesia remains a problem. Maybe the problem is not the agent. Stapleton et al. stated, "The plethora of new parenteral agents which the pharmaceutical companies have introduced over the past 20 years is not a reminder that we have not found the right drug but a reminder that we have not found the optimal mode of administration of perfectly adequate analgesic drugs."[53]

WHY NON-PATIENT-CONTROLLED TECHNIQUES FAIL

There are many non-patient-controlled techniques for postoperative analgesia following thoracic surgery. These include the use of opioids or nonopioid agents administered via intermittent bolus demand systems (oral; subcutaneous, SQ; intramuscular, IM; intravenous, IV); continuous infusions (SQ or IV); intercostal blockade (intercostal nerve blocks, continuous intercostal nerve blocks, intrapleural analgesia, cryoanalgesia); epidural or intrathecal techniques with local anesthetics; epidural or intrathecal narcotics; and transcutaneous electrical nerve stimulation (TENS). Given this large choice of analgesic agents and techniques, one would expect the perfect analgesic agent and/or technique to have been described by now.

Intermittent demand systems involve the use of oral or parenteral (IM or IV) narcotics. The inability to utilize the oral route because of altered gastrointestinal function caused parenteral opioids to become the most widely used method for providing postoperative analgesia. However, this system, utilizing opioid or nonopioid agents, has been shown to be inadequate. Reasons for this inadequacy derive from the technique of administration as well as the pharmacokinetics and pharmacodynamics of the drugs.

Figure 3–1 represents the cyclic character of conventional parenteral analgesic therapy, which has been described by Graves and colleagues,[54] illustrating potential delays between need and effect. A patient in pain requests medication by summoning a nurse, usually by a call button. This summons is answered by a ward clerk or nurse at some central location who, after determining the reason for the call, will find the patient's nurse provider. This nurse will either answer the patient via intercom or, preferably, see the patient, directly "screening" the patient by inquiring as to the type and severity of pain and evaluating the patient's sedation, respiratory status, "pain behavior," and the like. The nurse then checks the patient's medication record and orders to determine if another dose of analgesia is "warranted." Delays or perturbations in the cycle occur from the first step at which, for whatever reason (questionable stoicism, fear of addiction, embarrassment of "weakness," not wanting to bother the nurse with a nonemergent problem[55,56]), a patient may delay calling the nurse until the pain is unbearable and complications (e.g., splinting, tachycardia, hypertension, etc.) appear or worsen. The nurse's ability to respond will be a function of the number of nurses and

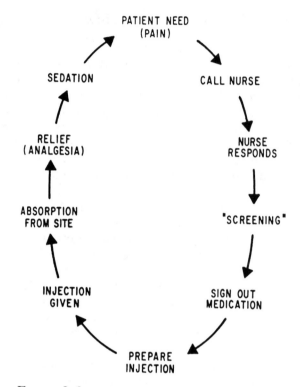

FIGURE 3–1. The cyclic character of conventional analgesic therapy. *(Reproduced, with permission, from Graves DA, Foster TS, Batenhorst RL, Bennett RL, Baumann TJ. Patient-controlled analgesia. Ann Intern Med 99:360–366, 1983)*

triage of nonemergent requests; and therefore, the number of analgesic injections received is directly proportional to nursing availability.[44] The delay in response has been estimated to be at least 30 minutes.[55] As was previously mentioned, results of the screening process and decision to provide analgesia to the patient are based on the education of the nursing staff and their misconceptions regarding appropriate analgesic use.

If the patient "passes the test," the nurse has to find the narcotics keys, obtain the medication from the narcotic lock box, sign out the medication, prepare the injection, administer the injection, and record narcotic given and wasted, usually in the presence of another nurse as required by hospital, state, and federal standards. This scenario is the same whether the analgesic is administered IV or IM. Onset and extent of analgesia are determined by the pharmacokinetic and pharmacodynamic profile of the agent, and effective opioid analgesia depends on obtaining and maintaining effective analgesic plasma levels of the opioid.

There is a direct relationship between postoperative analgesia and blood concentrations of meperidine.[57] Thus one can define a minimum effective analgesic concentration (MEAC) for an agent. For meperidine the concentration–response curve is so steep that as little as 0.05 µg/ml means the difference between analgesia and severe pain. Thus meperidine has a narrow effective concentration range.[57] If meperidine is given IM every 3 to 4 hours, then this narrow effective concentration and variable absorption results in meperidine blood levels exceeding the MEAC only 35% of the time.[57] Possible explanations include an up to five-fold interpatient variability between peak blood concentrations and the three- to seven-fold difference in time to peak concentrations when the same agent and dose is administered to a population of patients.[57,58] Hence, MEAC is highly variable between patients but more consistent within each individual patient over time.

MEAC is independent of method of drug delivery (IV vs IM).[57,58] Despite early evidence implying that elderly patients are more sensitive to opioids,[59] analgesic serum concentrations of meperidine appear to be independent of age.[60] Also, there is no scientific evidence for the calculation of analgesic dose based on sex,[59–62] body weight, or surface area.[59,63] Although blood analgesic concentration must remain in the range of MEAC for effective analgesia, in the absence of elimination abnormalities, individual pharmacokinetic variations (in volume of distribution, distribution, and elimination) between patients do not explain the three- to four-fold variations in analgesic concentrations.[60–62] Nevertheless, changes in volume of distribution, distribution rate, metabolism, and elimination may result in intrapatient changes in MEAC.[52]

Pharmacodynamic factors may be more important. Endogenous and exogenously administered opioids interact to alter MEAC and analgesic demand.[64,65] Postoperative analgesic requirements are inversely proportional to total preoperative CSF (endogenous) opioid levels.[64,65] These pharmacodynamic factors involve psychological variables (e.g., personality, anxiety, neuroticism, and coping skills) as measured on personality profiles. Analgesic requirement appears to be related to anxiety and neuroticism,[58,66] state anxiety,[67] and coping styles.[67] Hence inadequate analgesia is due to both individual fluctuating serum analgesic levels and significant individual variability in analgesic requirements.[57,58] Unfortunately, mathematical models involving these pharmacodynamic as well as pharmacokinetic variables are not solvable and, hence, it is difficult to predict individual analgesic requirements.

Conventional non-patient-controlled methods of postoperative analgesia ignore the patients' desire to retain control of their lives, which is completely lost to the physicians, nurses, dietary, housekeeping, and transport personnel when patients enter the hospital.[68] Not only is control over the outcome of the surgical procedure lost but control over privacy, mobility, and bodily functions is lost too. In general, patients prefer to control the timing of events and value predictability.[69,70] This control may be voluntarily abdicated if a patient perceives that, with another person in control, there is a greater chance of averting an unpleasant event.[71] In the cardiac intensive care population it has been shown that more information with little control has been equated with poor outcome while the best outcome is equated with a high degree of both information and participation in care.[72] Lack of control over an adverse event results in an increased perception of pain[73] and anxiety,[74] which itself increases the perception of pain. Having control results in the ability to tolerate more pain for a longer period of time.[70,75] Activity reduces stress and increases the ability to tolerate pain due to both the patient's control over the activity and its distracting ability.[76] Hence, in a situation in which the patient has only the power to request analgesics, loss of control is a pharmacodynamic factor that may increase the perception of pain and worsen the postoperative course.

Figure 3–2[77] describes the relationship between blood analgesic drug concentration and time. Effective analgesia will result only if one is able to exceed the MEAC and blood analgesic concentrations are within or above the patient's narrow therapeutic window (represented by the shaded area in Fig. 3–2). As the blood analgesic drug concentration increases, sedation and other side effects of the administered agent are seen. In Figure 3–2, bolus IM doses of opioids are shown as a solid line. After receiving an IM injection, onset of analgesia will not occur until the analgesic drug concentration is greater than or equal to the MEAC, and onset time is the time difference from injection to intersection of the concentration curve with the MEAC. The amplitude of the line is a function of the administered dose. Because the drug is only administered every 3 or 4 hours, large doses are required, resulting in high peak levels. The peak analgesic effect of morphine sulfate is 45 to 90 minutes after intramuscular injection,

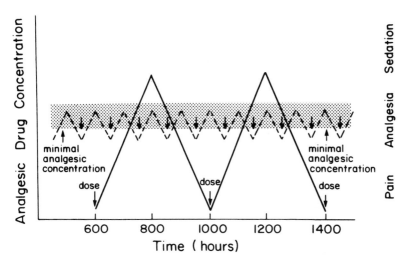

FIGURE 3–2.   Theoretical relation between analgesic drug concentration, dosing interval, and clinical response for PCA (---) and intramuscular opioid (___). Arrows pointing downward represent administration of patient-controlled or IM opioid doses. Reprinted with permission from the International Anesthesia Research Society *(Ferrante FM, Orav EJ, Rocco AG, Gallo J. A statistical model for pain in patient-controlled analgesia and conventional intramuscular regimens. Anesth Analg 67:457–461, 1987).*

and is somewhat less for the more lipophilic meperidine. Opioids produce a spectrum of effects, with analgesia occurring at lower serum concentrations than sedation. As the drug concentration exceeds the analgesic window sedation occurs (with an incidence as high as 46%[62]). As the analgesic agent is metabolized, blood concentration will decrease below the sedative level and the patient will awaken in a state of analgesia. The patient will remain analgesic until the concentration curve falls below the MEAC. The time period that the concentration curve remains at or above the MEAC is the duration of analgesic action of the agent. Concomitantly administered sedatives will enhance the sedative effect, so patients may not waken until the blood analgesic concentration is below the MEAC, thus the patient will awaken in pain. As the pain resumes, the patient will request another injection and will go through the same scenario as in Figure 3–1. Finally, even small changes in the MEAC may drastically shift the analgesic window such that similar doses of analgesics may not all result in analgesia.[78]

Intermittent, conventional bolus, IM administration of analgesics has been shown to be ineffective[1,3-5,7,80-84] due to this labor-intensive cyclical program of inadequate analgesia. In one study 59% of IM analgesic injections did not reach MEAC,[58] and in another study greater than 85% of attempted IM injections appeared to be subcutaneous.[79] These problems, coupled with the technique's limited dosage and time interval inflexibility, result in an inability to maintain constant serum concentrations and/or compensate for the wide individual variations in analgesic requirements.[84]

Compared to IM bolus administration, small intravenous bolus doses of opioids result in more effective analgesia with lower dosage requirements.[1] However, this method of analgesia is not practical because of the short duration of action, higher incidence of complications if higher doses are used to attempt to increase the duration of action, and high degree of labor intensity if a nurse–observer is used at each bedside.[85]

Understanding that acute pain has background and acute response components[26] led to the realization that patients require continuous analgesic coverage. The **fixed rate continuous intravenous infusion** of narcotics successfully provides analgesia in both postoperative and terminal patients.[1,86-89] Using the concept of MEAC, an approximation of the maintenance infusion rate may be estimated with the hope of keeping blood analgesic concentration within the therapeutic window (see Fig. 3–2). This system provides more stable therapeutic serum drug levels and lessens the frequency of inadequate analgesia because the patient is not waiting for an intermittent injection. The result is more stable analgesia and reduced nursing time.[84] However, the fixed rate continuous technique also has an onset delay of 3.3 to 5 times the half-life in order to reach 90% to 95% of steady state serum concentrations. These steady state drug concentrations may vary two-fold due to normal individual drug metabolism and elimination. Thus, inadequate steady state levels and inadequate analgesia may result.[84] Risk of accumulation of the agents resulting in undesirable side effects[80,86] may occur secondary to a normally wide range of drug clearances between different patients and within the same patient, variation in narcotic need, circadian variation in pain and pharmacokinetics,[90] and long half-lives of some of the agents. With the fixed rate continuous technique, the possibility of overdosing a patient exists when the rate is set to provide analgesia for acute (transient) response pain.[84] Finally, despite better analgesia, continuous infusion may be inferior to intermittent bolus administration due to the more rapid development of tolerance.[91]

A continuous infusion technique in which the maintenance rate was varied according to the patient's complaints has been described.[81] Its efficacy was confirmed in comparison with conventional IM therapy.[81] However, there were problems with both the onset time and acute response pain.[84] The **modified, variable rate, continuous infusion** technique[50] corrected these deficits with a bolus loading dose to achieve a rapid onset of analgesia with blood analgesic concentrations rising to the therapeutic window, and a variable infusion rate titrated to a minimal, safe analgesic level based on the patient's reports of pain. Supplemental IV narcotics were used for breakthrough or acute response pain to compensate for sudden increases in MEAC and the therapeutic window. In postoperative patients this technique resulted in better analgesia, decreased amount of narcotics used, more stable drug concentrations, and the ability to rapidly titrate the infusion to compensate for changes in pain states. This technique also resulted in better respiratory mechanics and fewer side effects. Most notably, there was a lack of respiratory depression, hemodynamic instability, dose-escalation secondary to tolerance, addiction, and physical dependence.[50,81,84]

Problems with this technique may occur when MEAC and estimates of volume of distribution and clearance are utilized to calculate loading dose and maintenance infusion rates, as there may be at least a two-fold variation in effective doses between patients.[57,58,84]

Regional anesthesia techniques, such as peripheral nerve, epidural, or intrathecal blocks (with local anesthetic agents or opioids) have been shown to be useful for analgesia in the postoperative thoracic surgical patient. A detailed discussion of the indications, contraindications, efficacy, side effects, complications, and comparative studies may be found in other chapters in this book or a recent review of pain management in the critically ill.[52] Of these techniques intercostal blockade, epidural local anesthetic block, and epidural or intrathecal opioids may be the most useful in this patient population. All of these techniques are invasive and all require specialized skills and experience to perform.

TENS, although controversial, may be effective in managing postoperative background and acute response pain with reduced incidence of atelectasis and ileus and increased patient mobility.[92-98] There are virtually no side effects with this technique, which some have found useful, either alone or as an adjunct to reduced doses of opioids.[97,98] TENS units stimulate the afferent nervous system via cutaneous electrodes. Two theories of action are that analgesia is produced via electrical interference with the spinal transmission of pain impulses[99] and that electrical stimulation increases serotonin to centrally inhibit pain signal transmission.[100] Electrode placement appears to be the major problem. The technique does not appear to be effective in patients with preexisting chronic opioid use,[101] and its efficacy has been challenged in chronic pain management.[102]

PATIENT-CONTROLLED ANALGESIA: HISTORY AND EARLY STUDIES

The concept of a "patient-controlled" analgesic system utilizing subanesthetic doses of potent anesthetic agents is not new. As early as 1847 Simpson utilized subanesthetic concentrations of an inhalational agent (chloroform) to induce intermittent inhalational analgesia in a parturient. Although this was "demand analgesia," it is questionable whether this soaked towel method was self-administered. Beginning in the 1930s, self-administered inhalational (patient-controlled) analgesia became a popular method for analgesia during labor. Utilizing the Cyprane[103] and Duke[104] inhalers with trichlorethylene, patients were able to self-administer analgesia. Strapped onto the forearm (Cyprane) or with a patient-activated on/off switch (Duke) the patient inhaled trichlorethylene until analgesia or sedation was achieved and either the forearm and mask fell away from her face (Cyprane) or her finger relaxed to turn off the switch (Duke) and terminate the gas flow. When the patient awoke the technique was repeated as necessary. These trichlorethylene inhalers fell out of use because of complications of trichlorethylene, nonphysiologic analgesia, and anecdotal reports of complications resulting from inappropriate or not "self-administered" use. The technique was frequently nonphysiologic, as the time period from onset to peak of contraction was often shorter than the onset of analgesia. With the release of methoxyflurane in the 1960s, the Penthrane Analgizer™ and Penthrane Whistle™ were widely utilized for patient-controlled inhalational analgesia during labor and delivery.[105,106] Again, problems regarding delayed onset of analgesia and the acceptance of epidural analgesia led to their disappearance.

Following surgery, self-administered methoxyflurane with an Abbott Analgizer™ increased postoperative vital capacity with efficacy equal to 10 mg of IM morphine, without morphine-induced depression of alveolar ventilation.[107] Self-administered, patient-controlled inhalational analgesia with regulated mixtures of nitrous oxide and oxygen are still utilized for the treatment of acute response pain.[108] However, as nitrous oxide diffuses into and enlarges gas containing cavities, the danger of converting a simple pneumothorax into a tension pneumothorax in the event of a non- or partially functioning chest tube limits its use following thoracic surgery.

Combining the finding that small intravenous bolus doses of narcotic analgesics produced greater analgesia at lower doses than IM administration[1] and the concept of patient control,[85] Sechzer developed patient-controlled intravenous analgesia (PCA). He hypothesized that patient's analgesic needs, as demonstrated by pressing a button to demand and/or deliver analgesia, would continue until the analgesic threshold was reached and this would be a measure of pain.[85] In 1968 Sechzer reported a study on postoperative analgesia in 20 patients (including 6 postthoracotomy) in whom he measured the postoperative analgesic response to small intravenous bolus doses of opioids (morphine sulfate or meperidine HCI) administered by a nurse–observer on demand.[16] He found that postoperative pain and, therefore, analgesic demand was cyclical, varied considerably among subjects, and, in the absence of complications, was consistent within each patient. This "analgesic-demand system" improved analgesia with less total opioid use but was too labor intensive to be clinically useful.

In 1970, Forrest et al., reported the successful use of a patient-operated demand analgesic device with reliable "fail-safe" features in 30 patients, finding good patient and physician acceptance.[109] This Demand Dropmaster™ automatically dispensed a present volume of intravenous analgesic agent on demand via a patient-activated button. Safety features included measurement and limits for individual and total doses, and a timer that defined a period after a requested dose during which the device would not deliver additional doses (lock-out interval). In 1971, Sechzer reported his experience with an automated patient-controlled analgesic-demand device.[110] It was a successful system for achieving postoperative analgesia using less narcotics than would have been expected under scheduled regimens.

The first comparison of a demand analgesia apparatus with conventional intramuscular analgesic therapy was by Keeri-Szanto.[111,112] The Demanalg™ device decreased the incidence of "substantial" postoperative pain from between 20% and 40% to less than 5%. When this demand analgesia group was returned to standard intramuscular analgesic therapy, the incidence of inadequate analgesia increased to 30% despite increased doses of opioids.

The first commercially available intravenous patient-controlled analgesic device, the Cardiff Palliator, was developed at the Welch National School of Medicine in 1976.[113] This device proved effective for postoperative analgesia using a variety of analgesic agents.[114–117] However, in one study, the demand button was deemed too difficult to operate, and the authors found this apparatus too expensive and time-consuming.[118]

A major advance in patient-controlled analgesia therapy occurred with the development of the on-demand analgesic computer, ODAC™, which includes subjective and objective patient feedback.[119,120] With ODAC™, the patient is able to interact directly with the computer via an audio tape cassette, and a variable background infusion may be administered based on the patient's demands over the previous 16 minutes. In addition, the dosage delivered by ODAC™ is limited by the patient's respiratory rate. In clinical studies there was no evidence of drug accumulation or tolerance with this device.[119]

Tamsen and colleagues used the Pharmacia Prominject™, a programmable pump, in their pharmacokinetic and pharmacodynamic studies.[62,64,82,121,122] Despite the four- to six-fold interpatient variability in analgesic requirements and analgesic drug concentrations, these individual PCA patients were able to maintain relatively constant plasma drug concentrations.[82] The mean postoperative analgesic requirements were 2.7 ± 1.1 mg/hr for morphine and 26 ± 10 mg/hr for meperidine.[82] Patient complaints included sedation and dry mouth.[82]

In a series of studies at the University of Kentucky, utilizing the Demanalg™ PCA pump for postoperative analgesia, Bennett et al. demonstrated adequate analgesia with minimal sedation,[123,124] an average morphine requirement of 1.7 mg/hr with a ten-fold interpatient variation,[125] and a circadian variation in postoperative analgesic requirements.[126]

PCA: MODES AND CURRENTLY AVAILABLE PUMPS

There are four modes of PCA: bolus demand, bolus demand with constant infusion, infusion demand, and bolus demand with variable infusion.[127] Bolus demand and bolus demand with constant infusion pumps are currently commercially available. Infusion demand and bolus demand with variable infusion pumps are experimental.

With **bolus demand,** preset doses are delivered on patient demand depending on the maximum dose and lockout interval. **Bolus demand with constant infusion** is a system in which a basal infusion is utilized in addition to bolus demand. Theoretically, this system should avoid the decreases in blood analgesic concentration during sleep. **Infusion demand** is similar to bolus demand mode except that the patient's demands vary only the infusion rate. Finally, **bolus demand with variable infusion** allows for bolus demands and varies the infusion rate based on the number and frequency of previous bolus demands.

At the present time a number of PCA infusion devices are commercially available. Most are mechanical, electrical infusion devices with locking safeguards in which the physician or nurse sets the bolus loading dose, incremental dose, lock-out interval, total dose over a given time period, and, in some, a basal infusion rate. There is one small, portable, relatively inexpensive, nonelectric, nonprogrammable, hydrostatic device also available. The attributes of the numerous available PCA devices are described in detail in several excellent publications,[128–132] and will not be described here.

PCA: THEORETICAL BENEFITS

Theoretical benefits of PCA include a more physiologic, rapid response, patient-controlled analgesic system, with more consistent therapeutic blood analgesic levels. This results in decreased pain or painful time periods, decreased anxiety, decreased total analgesic use, decreased complications (sedation, respiratory depression, etc.), and decreased nursing time. It also imparts a sense of control to the patients over their lives.

PCA: COMPARATIVE STUDIES WITH OTHER TECHNIQUES

Since the first comparison of PCA and conventional IM analgesia by Keeri-Szanto,[111] a great deal has been written regarding PCA including several reviews.[54,130–134] Unfortunately, there are few controlled, randomized, double-blinded studies and even fewer concerning postthoracotomy pain. Many parallels may be drawn from earlier studies.

In 1984, Finley, Keeri-Szanto, and Boyd compared PCA to conventional IM postoperative analgesia in nonthoracotomy patients.

PCA improved early postoperative mobilization and cooperation with physical therapy regimens in addition to decreasing postoperative hospital stay by 22%.[135] Various nonthoracic studies have shown that PCA offers improved analgesia over conventional IM narcotic analgesia and some show decreased sedation.[54,111,121,124,126,136-141] Some also report a lower incidence of nocturnal sleep disturbance and greater physical activity.[120,126,142-144] Although some studies show no difference in analgesia between PCA and IM groups, one indicated that the IM group had a treatable cycle of pain every 5.3 hours which was not seen in the PCA group.[77] One reason for this apparent discrepancy is that some patients do not titrate PCA to complete analgesia.[77,139] Rather, they titrate to expected pain and hence, to what they believe as possible analgesia.[77] Moreover, some patients may prefer to tolerate mild pain in order to avoid the sedative effects of narcotics.[123,145] Finally, some studies of equivalent analgesia with PCA versus IM administration alter another variable between the groups (e.g., availability of nursing staff,[146] different medications,[147] and supplemental IV bolus narcotics[148]) and thus, their stated results may not be applicable.

Early studies indicate that PCA patients require less narcotics than patients treated with conventional IM regimens,[124] even though the latter patients received less satisfactory analgesia. More recent studies show either no difference in total amount of analgesic utilized[136,140,148,149] or greater total amount of narcotic utilized with PCA.[84,136,139,150,151] White reported that PCA patients require less medication for the first 48 hours postoperatively than patients on IM regimens, but tend to require parenteral narcotics for a longer time postoperatively.[152]

Most studies comparing PCA with IM regimens report no difference in the incidence of respiratory depression, nausea, vomiting, or pruritus.[136,139,150] However, in a study comparing IM morphine with PCA fentanyl after upper abdominal surgery, a greater number of PCA patients had mildly elevated carbon dioxide levels.[147] Tamsen has reported respiratory depression in two elderly hypovolemic patients which was corrected with fluid administration.[82] The details of these cases leave some questions about whether these were cause and effect. Other studies show improvement in postoperative pulmonary function, fewer respiratory complications, and faster recovery of minute ventilation with PCA.[82,153] These improvements result in a lower incidence of postoperative fevers and earlier discharge from the hospital.[140]

PCA allows patients some control over their lives in a situation in which most control and decisions are surrendered to others. Control means that the patient no longer needs to convince others to deliver analgesic therapy and is able to titrate the analgesic to the level of pain and sedation they are willing to accept.[68] This may explain why PCA patients sometimes require less medication and report better analgesia than those on conventional therapies.[82,124,136] Increased initial use of analgesics with subsequent decreased levels may indicate the patient initially exerting or testing his or her control.[124,154] Finally, control with PCA allows the patient to dose themselves to their own expectations of analgesia, remain satisfied with the PCA technique, and yet claim pain scores of 2 to 3 (0–10 scale).[77,155]

Following posterolateral thoracotomy, Lange and colleagues reported decreased narcotic utilization and a decreased incidence of postoperative fevers and pulmonary complications in patients on PCA compared to IM narcotics.[156] Wang et al, evaluated PCA versus IM therapy postthoracotomy and reported decreased pain, decreased nocturnal sleep disturbances, and a greater ratio of postoperative to preoperative FVC in the PCA group.[157]

PCA did not compare favorably with the modified variable rate continuous infusion of morphine sulfate in critically ill patients, presumably due to a lack of background analgesia.[158] Specifically, PCA failed to provide analgesia after both acute burn injury and when used as a step down device following continuous infusion. This was despite dosage adjustments, greater total amount of morphine infused, more supplemental boluses of morphine, and supplemental anxiolytics while on PCA. Only the PCA group complained of agitation, pain on awakening, nightmares, insomnia, and nausea. These complaints disappeared when the patients returned to continuous infusion and achieved more consistent background analgesia.

Intravenous PCA (IV-PCA) has also been compared with epidural techniques involving epidural local analgesics and opioids. White et al. found that, IV fentanyl provided equivalent postoperative analgesia to epidural bupivacaine.[159] Comparisons with epidural narcotics appear less promising for IV-PCA. Epidural opioids provided better analgesia than IV-PCA opioids following cesarean section, total joint replacement, and total abdominal hysterectomy.[160-163] After the first 16 hours, analgesia was similar in the cesarean section study.[160] The epidural groups had a higher incidence of pruritus,[160,161,163] but there was no difference in time to mobilization, eating, or hospital discharge.[160,162] Although there was a significantly lower minimum respiratory rate in the epidural group, no treatment of respiratory depression was needed.[163] Comparing single bolus epidural and IV-PCA morphine following C-section,[139,150] epidural morphine provided superior analgesia for at least the first 16 hours.[150] PCA caused more sedation while epidural narcotics induced more pruritus. The epidural groups required more supplemental IV analgesics. Mild pain was tolerated in the IV-PCA groups and both IV-PCA and epidural groups preferred their therapy to conventional IM analgesics. In another study comparing IV-PCA morphine, epidural morphine, and epidural morphine plus bupivacaine following abdominal surgery, PCA and epidural morphine patients had equivalent analgesia, ability to cough, and rate pressure products.[164] The epidural morphine plus bupivacaine group was superior in all three parameters, but there was no difference in time to bowel function, duration of hospitalization, or frequency or intensity of complications. Epidural morphine infusion patients had shorter hospital stays than IV-PCA morphine patients following knee reconstruction.[165] Despite equivalent analgesia, epidural opioids and not IV-PCA suppressed norepinephrine and cortisol response following lower extremity revascularization.[166]

Patients receiving epidural fentanyl infusions following thoracic surgery had superior analgesia at rest and with cough compared to patients receiving bolus IV-PCA morphine.[167] However, the epidural group also had a higher incidence of pruritus. Both groups had similar postoperative decreases in vital capacity, incidences of sedation, nausea, and vomiting, and mild increases in $PaCO_2$. After thoracic surgery, patients apparently do not utilize IV-PCA to achieve complete analgesia but rather to reach an individually derived level of expected comfort.[168]

PCA PLUS CONTINUOUS INFUSION TECHNIQUES

With bolus PCA devices there were problems with loss of analgesia during sleep due to a lack of background analgesia. Some patients receiving longer acting analgesic agents via PCA for acute response pain were then "overdosed" during periods of background pain. Other patients receiving the newer, shorter acting analgesic agents required frequent dosing.

PCA infusion devices that incorporate bolus PCA plus continuous (background or basal) infusion capabilities were developed to address these problems. Utilizing this technique, relationships between blood concentration and analgesic response (MEAC) were developed for fentanyl[169] and sufentanil.[170] IV-PCA was efficacious with both these agents.[169,170] The combination of PCA plus continuous (background) infusion was found superior by 36% to 47% of patients when compared to prior experience with conventional postoperative analgesic therapy.[171] This continuous plus on-demand bolus technique with shorter acting agents was less sedating than conventional IM therapy with longer acting agents.[172] Following thoracotomy, IV-PCA plus continuous infusion was preferred by patients to conventional IM regimens.[173] High doses of analgesics were used with both techniques, and there was no statistically significant difference in the few side effects including respiratory depression.[173]

A comparison of IV-PCA plus background infusion, IM opioids, intercostal block, and epidural opioids following upper abdominal surgery demonstrated similar pain scores (when IM narcotics were administered on demand) and no difference in chest x-ray, PEF, or respiratory rate.[137] However, the PCA plus continuous infusion group had a slightly elevated $PaCO_2$ and a greater percentage of patients rating their analgesia as good. Following cesarean section, PCA plus continuous infusion was comparable to epidural morphine in analgesia, time to activity (sitting, ambulating), time to tolerating clear fluids, and hospital discharge.[174] Pruritus and alarms from apnea monitors occurred only in the epidural group. Following thoracotomy, PCA plus continuous infusion was as effective as a combination of epidural bupivacaine and sufentanil in providing analgesia, but neither was superior in preserving vital capacity postoperatively.[175]

Finally, does PCA plus continuous "basal" infusion offer an improvement over PCA alone? In a series of postoperative studies, PCA plus continuous infusion resulted in better analgesia,[176–179] fewer sleep disturbances,[176] less awakening with pain,[176] and more patient satisfaction[176,178] than PCA alone. Less nausea and vomiting was seen in one study[176] and more in another.[177] Sedation was greater with PCA plus continuous infusion in one study,[178] but no difference in sedation was noted between the two groups in another.[180] Other studies demonstrate no benefit in adding a continuous infusion to PCA therapy and claim increased drug utilization without an increase in analgesia[181–184] or decrease in the number of patient demands.[181] PCA plus continuous infusion may alter the blood concentration–analgesic response relationship[182] and, hence, may reduce the inherent safety of PCA.[184]

POSTOPERATIVE IV-PCA THERAPY: REQUIREMENTS FOR EFFECTIVE THERAPY

Effective postoperative analgesic therapy with IV-PCA has been described in detail by White.[131] Its success depends on an understanding of the concept (see Fig. 3–1 and 3–2) by the physicians, nurses, patients, and their families, and the correct choice of analgesic agent and dosing parameters. Possible complications of the technique must also be understood.

Physicians and nurses need to understand the benefits of analgesia, the ability of patients to care for themselves and dose themselves to an analgesic state, and the importance to the patients of being in control. The PCA device needs to be explained to the patients and their families preoperatively, when they are not under duress. Patients should be told to utilize the device to avoid severe pain, without the expectation of complete analgesia and to use the PCA device prophylactically, prior to painful activity, procedures, or treatment, to avoid acute exacerbations of pain. Patients should be informed that the goals of PCA are to achieve analgesia with the minimal possible dose to avoid sedation and to maximize the analgesic interval to allow for uninterrupted sleep.

POSTOPERATIVE IV-PCA THERAPY: DOSING PARAMETERS

Dosing parameters set by the physician include: choice of drug, loading dose, incremental bolus dose per demand, lockout interval, maximum dose per unit time, and basal or continuous infusion rate. The characteristics of the ideal analgesic agent were discussed earlier. In the absence of an ideal agent, choose the agent best suited for the particular situation. Drugs of intermediate duration of action (morphine or meperidine) have been preferred in most clinical trials. The shortest acting agents (alfentanil, sufentanil) may be successfully utilized, but usually require a continuous infusion to decrease the frequency of demands. Analgesic ceiling effects of mixed opioids tend to limit their use. It is not just the analgesic agent, but also the technique of administration utilized for the individual agent that is important to a successful analgesic regimen.[185] Guidelines for the use of opioid analgesics as well as a suggested regimen have been described by White and are listed in Table 3–1.[131]

TABLE 3–1. Guidelines for Bolus Doses and Lockout Intervals
for Parenteral Analgesics When Using PCA

Drug	Bolus Dose (mg or μg)	Lockout Interval (min)
Agonists		
Morphine	0.5–3.0	5–20
Methadone	0.5–3.0	10–20
Hydromorphone	0.1–0.5	5–15
Meperidine	5–30	5–15
Fentanyl	15–75	3–10
Sufentanil	2–10	3–10
Agonist–Antagonist		
Pentazocine	5–30	5–15
Nalbuphine	1–5	5–15
Buprenorphine	0.03–0.2	5–20

(*Reproduced with permission from White PF. Patient-controlled analgesia: A new approach to the management of postoperative pain. Semin Anesth 4:255–266, 1985*)

Unless analgesia has been achieved by loading the patient with the analgesic agent intraoperatively, a loading intravenous bolus dose of 2 to 10 mg morphine or 25 to 100 mg meperidine over 15 to 30 minutes is recommended in adults to achieve analgesia. This loading dose should be administered in the post anesthesia care unit before the patient begins using the PCA device. Although a milligram per kilogram approach to analgesia is not recommended for continued use, 0.05 mg/kg for morphine and 0.5 mg/kg for meperidine are good starting points for a loading dose in a nondebilitated or compromised adult. This titrated loading dose is highly patient dependent and may be repeated every 10 to 20 minutes until analgesia is achieved, or for breakthrough pain once PCA therapy has begun. As the agent is titrated until the patient receives analgesia, milligram per kilogram dosing may be justified as a starting point.

Once they are sufficiently recovered from the effects of anesthesia and able to comprehend the self-administration of analgesics, patients may be started on PCA therapy by giving them the "button or control pad." Beginning with 1 to 2 mg bolus doses of morphine or 10 to 20 mg bolus doses of meperidine, the dose is increased by 25% to 50% increments for inadequate analgesia until a satisfactory dose is found, or decreased by 25% to 50% in the case of unwanted side effects (excessive sedation, dizziness, respiratory compromise). The dose may be increased or a continuous infusion added to allow a longer time interval between doses for sleep. Using this protocol, White found a wide variability in individual morphine requirements with a range of median hourly requirements of 1.1 to 2.6 mg/hr in patients following major surgery.[131] Seventy-one percent of these patients reported a lack of significant discomfort and 29% noted mild to moderate pain during the study.

With noncompromised nonpediatric patients, without a continuous basal infusion, I recommend the following regimen:

Agent	Loading Dose	Incremental Dose	Lockout Interval	4-Hour Maximum
Morphine	0.05 mg/kg	0.02 mg/kg	6–10 min	30 mg
Meperidine	0.5 mg/kg	0.2 mg/kg	10–15 min	300 mg

When using a continuous basal infusion, the same loading dose and 4-hour maximum may be used, but the incremental morphine dose is changed to 0.5 to 0.75 mg, lockout interval of 8 to 10 minutes, and a continuous infusion rate of 0.015 mg/kg/hr. The infusion rate can be increased by 30% at night. These regimens should be evaluated for efficacy prior to the patient's discharge from the PACU, 2 to 4 hours after return to the ward, and several times during the day. As there is no relationship between MEAC and body weight, the use of a dose based on body weight represents only a starting point. There should be medical follow-up by physicians, nurses, and/or pharmacists as to efficacy and side effects.

POSTOPERATIVE IV-PCA THERAPY: SPECIAL POPULATION GROUPS

One would expect patients with high postoperative pain levels to utilize more narcotics on PCA than patients with less pain.[186] With PCA, anxious, depressed, and negative thinking patients tend to make a greater number of drug demands, however, they do not necessarily use more narcotics than less distressed patients because of the lockout interval.[186] In addition, different surgical procedures may interact with patients' characteristics to complicate the patients' perception of analgesia.[187,188] Four populations of patients cause increased concern when managing acute postoperative pain with PCA: older patients, chronic pain patients, substance abusers, and children.

Controversy exists regarding the effect of age on analgesic requirements. In spite of the fact that serum concentrations of opioids are independent of age,[60] the elderly have a decreased requirement for analgesic agents.[59] This has been shown in their decreased narcotic requirement while using PCA.[189-191] Given the same dose of opioids, the elderly have higher plasma levels than the young,[192] owing to decreased drug clearance with age and greater fraction of unbound "free" drug. This may result in a higher incidence of side effects. There may be pharmacodynamic changes at the opioid receptors resulting in an increased response.[193] The elderly may have different expectations of analgesia, thus they may use less narcotic via PCA, and yet accept less satisfactory pain relief.[77,190,191]

Although one might expect increased postoperative opioid use from chronic pain patients, this has not been demonstrated. However, chronic pain patients tend to accept higher postoperative pain scores,[194] which may serve as another demonstration that patients titrate PCA to their individual pain expectations.[77]

Substance abuse patients also pose a difficult problem. Few doubt that substance abuse patients experience acute postoperative pain, however, there are questions regarding their possible abuse of PCA and, therefore, its efficacy.[195] Problems of tolerance, habituation, and dependent or avoidance coping strategies complicate the use of PCA in this population. Substance abuse patients can achieve safe and adequate PCA without prolonged use, however, they require larger narcotic doses and sometimes require a basal infusion.[196]

Pediatric postoperative pain management has historically been neglected and felt to be unnecessary by some. Few or no narcotic analgesics are often ordered for children having the same procedures as adults, and children receive a smaller percentage of what is ordered.[197,198] The effect of postthoracotomy pain in a child is no different than in an adult. Respiratory dysfunction secondary to pain is manifest as splinting, diminished tidal volume, elevated $PaCO_2$, and increased alveolar-to-arterial oxygen difference.[199] Increased oxygen consumption in children may render these effects more significant, and they can be reversed with adequate analgesia.[199] Although it is often difficult to estimate the amount of pain in children, long-term consequences of inadequate analgesia make treatment of this problem imperative.[200]

IV-PCA has been shown to be effective in children as young as 11 years of age following major (including thoracic) surgery.[201-203]

Good analgesia, few side effects, and patient preference over prior regimens has been documented. Similar to adults,[124] pediatric patients tended to use more narcotics for the first postoperative day, however, total narcotic utilization over the postoperative period was less with IV-PCA than conventional IM regimens.[201] After pectus excavatum repair, PCA resulted in better analgesia than conventional IM regimens, but required 1.5 to 3 times the amount of drug without difference in side effects.[204] This probably reveals underdosing of patients in the IM group. IV-PCA has been used in patients as young as 5 years of age following general, orthopedic, and thoracic surgery with excellent analgesia, minimal sedation, and no evidence of respiratory depression.[205,206] Thirty-four percent of patients incurred minor agent-related side effects (constipation, pruritus, nausea, or vomiting) while 5.3% had problems with understanding the pump or the concept of PCA, resulting in overmedication with sedation.[205] This technique allows for long-term analgesic therapy without tolerance or dependence.[207] Both PCA and PCA plus continuous infusion provide better analgesia and more normal sleeping cycles than IM therapy without increasing the amount of narcotics utilized, sedation, or other drug related side effects.[201,208] In addition, patient control of analgesic therapy is especially important in children and adolescents.[201,203]

Pediatric PCA regimens use weight-based dosing as a starting point. Rodgers and colleagues suggest morphine (1 mg/ml), with a loading dose of 0.05 to 0.10 mg/kg, incremental bolus of 0.025 to 0.05 mg/kg, lockout interval of 10 to 15 minutes, and a 4-hour maximum limit of 0.1 to 0.2 mg/kg.[201] At the Children's National Medical Center Broadman employs lower parameters with incremental doses of 0.02 mg/kg and a 15 minute lockout period.[203]

COMPLICATIONS OF IV-PCA

Potential complications of PCA may be divided into four categories: adverse reactions and side effects, mechanical problems, operator-related problems, and user-related problems. Adverse reactions and side effects of this technique are, for the most part, based on the side effects of the agents utilized and include respiratory depression, sedation, pruritus, nausea, vomiting, allergic reactions, tolerance, and the like. Other potential problems such as entrainment of air, thrombophlebitis, IV disconnections, infiltration, and hemorrhage are possible complications of IV access. Table 3–2 lists operator errors, pa-

TABLE 3–2.   Summary of Problems That Can Occur During
Patient-controlled Analgesia (PCA) Therapy

> Operator errors
> > Misprogramming PCA device
> > Failure to clamp or unclamp tubing
> > Improperly loading syringe or cartridge
> > Inability to respond to safety alarms
> > Misplacing PCA pump key
>
> Patient errors
> > Failure to understand PCA therapy
> > Misunderstanding PCA pump device
> > Intentional analgesic abuse
>
> Mechanical problems
> > Failure to deliver on demand
> > Cracked drug vials or syringes
> > Defective one-way valve at "Y" connector
> > Faulty alarm system
> > Malfunctions (*e.g.*, lock)

(Reproduced with permission from White PF. Mishaps with patient-controlled analgesia. Anesthesiology 66:81–83, 1987)

tient errors, and mechanical problems.[209] Fortunately, the incidence of problems with PCA is small, and this is probably due to the inherent safety of self-administered analgesic therapy.

Of all adverse effects, the one that frightens providers into undertreatment is respiratory depression. Yet, there is a low incidence of respiratory depression with postoperative PCA therapy. Following upper abdominal surgery, a greater percentage of PCA patients have elevated capillary carbon dioxide levels than patients receiving IM or epidural opioids.[147] However, postoperative respiratory function in PCA patients does not differ significantly from conventional IM regimen patients[111,147,171] and obese PCA-treated patients have been noted to have improved pulmonary function postoperatively.[153] Moreover, following major surgical procedures, PCA patients have maintained normal arterial blood gases.[82,159] Reported cases of severe respiratory depression are anecdotal because the system has its own negative feedback control. If a patient receives a large dose of narcotic via PCA and the blood analgesic concentration exceeds the therapeutic window into the sedation range (Fig. 3–2), the patient will be too sedated to demand another dose. This situation will continue until this "overdose" blood concentration decreases and falls below the sedation threshold where only analgesia remains. This sedation should be noted by the staff and the incremental dose decreased. Hence, by a negative feedback mechanism patients will be "protected" against dosing themselves to respiratory depression. If, however, someone else controls the demand button on the PCA device (parent or spouse), then this negative feedback internal safety feature of PCA is lost.[210]

Patients at risk for respiratory depression include the very young, elderly, debilitated, and those with preexisting respiratory insufficiency. Respiratory depression manifesting as hypercarbia and hypoventilation has been reported in a patient with sleep apnea syndrome receiving PCA with basal infusion.[211] Others have pointed to the potential danger of continuous basal infusion distorting the inherent safety of PCA.[212] Setting the basal infusion rate at a level less than that needed for complete analgesia (MEAC) has been suggested to avoid this problem.[212]

Severe respiratory depression secondary to operator and patient errors has been described,[209] as have alleged machine errors resulting in respiratory arrest.[213] Other machine related problems such as pump reactivation by reinsertion of a power plug and problems with antireflux valves have also been described.[214,215]

The development of tolerance requiring larger and larger doses of narcotic analgesics poses a special problem. Although this may occur, IV-PCA has been utilized for prolonged periods without development of tolerance.[207] The discontinuation of PCA or any opioid delivery system after prolonged use may result in withdrawal symptoms. This may be treated by tapering the narcotics (IV or PO) or with clonidine. Some consider a history of substance abuse to be a contraindication to PCA because of possible problems with patient tampering[216] or excessive use.[195] However, others have successfully utilized PCA in this population.[196]

IV-PCA: COST EFFECTIVENESS

IV-PCA is not inexpensive. In a clinical study of burn patients it was found to be 4.6 times more expensive in hospital costs (pumps, tubing, agents) per day than the modified variable rate continuous infusion technique.[158] However, this study did not measure either the costs related to nursing time or the possible costs associated with loss of patient control, hospital stay, and the like, nor did the study account for the fact that the continuous infusion pumps were provided free of charge. Ready has examined the economics of IV-PCA therapy[217] and found no statistically significant difference in hospital costs (equipment, drugs, and nursing time) between IV-PCA and IM regimens. He further showed that Seattle area hospital collections exceeded their IV-PCA costs (in 1990), even in the face of a 60% collection rate, and there was a nursing-time savings of 33 min/patient/day with PCA. Because of shrinking health care dollars, the ability to obtain reimbursement for PCA equipment, agents, and services may be limited. However, improved postoperative analgesia, improved pulmonary function,[153] decreased postoperative fevers, and fewer chest X-ray changes following thoracotomy[156] reduce postoperative complications and make PCA cost-effective at least in comparison to conventional IM narcotic analgesia. To this end, Rao and colleagues demonstrated an average savings of 4.3 in-hospital days over DRG days allowable. This may be invalid on the basis of patient selection and no patient control group.

NEW CONCEPTS IN PCA

New concepts in patient-controlled analgesia involve the use of patient-controlled epidural analgesia (PCEA), subcutaneous PCA (SQ-PCA), sublingual PCA (SL-PCA), cerebral ventricular PCA (V-PCA), and patient-controlled sedation (PCS). PCEA with continuous plus on demand capabilities has been recommended in the treatment of postoperative pain because it combines constant analgesia with the possibility of individualized treatment.[219] However, some have shown no significant benefit of PCEA with basal infusion over bolus PCEA alone.[220] They claim that PCEA plus basal infusion utilizes more narcotics without changes in postoperative analgesia, side effects, or recovery time. They also note that tolerance occurs more rapidly in the PCEA patients with the basal infusion. Bolus PCEA fentanyl plus continuous epidural bupivacaine infusion utilizes less narcotic than continuous epidural infusions of both bupivacaine and fentanyl, but provides equal postoperative analgesia.[221]

Analgesia depends on the attainment of adequate drug concentrations at the receptors, irrespective of the method of administration. IV-PCA with fentanyl results in a faster onset of analgesia than PCEA because of more rapid achievement of MEAC.[222] However, when alfentanil is used, the onset of analgesia is identical with both methods of administration.[223] PCEA requires less narcotic than IV-PCA for equivalent analgesia.[223–225] Some claim greater analgesia with PCEA, but only on the first postoperative day.[226] Some studies demonstrate no differences in opioid-related side effects with either technique[226] (especially respiratory depression[227]) while others show more oxygen desaturations with PCEA utilizing alfentanil.[223] Pruritus is more common with PCEA.[227] Urinary retention requiring catheterization is more frequent with PCEA, but only when a combination of local anesthetic and narcotic is utilized.[227] When narcotics alone are used following nephrectomy, PCEA results in earlier removal of the Foley catheter, a lower incidence of pneumonias, and earlier discharge from the hospital than with IV-PCA.[228]

SQ-PCA appears to be as effective as IV-PCA except that it does not require IV access.[229,230] It has been used in the ambulatory care of patients with advanced diseases[231] via simple and inexpensive infusion pumps.[232] This technique requires larger doses of opioids than IV-PCA.[229,230] SL-PCA has been described in the literature,[233] as has a device for V-PCA for patients with intractable pain.[234] V-PCA requires only small doses of narcotic for prolonged analgesia.

The concept of patient-controlled sedation (PCS) or patient-controlled anxiolysis (PCAx) is a logical extension of the concept of PCA. That is, patients should be able to more effectively dose themselves to an anxiolytic state with an on-demand, patient-controlled system rather than with intermittent nurse- or physician-controlled conventional regimens. The need for such a system is obvious, at least in the intensive care situation, where concern for the patient's psychological or mental health frequently takes a second priority. Fear and anxiety have been reported in as many as 70% of ICU patients.[235] Patients report feelings of loss of control, fear of physical harm, and sense of impending doom.[236] Loper and colleagues described a midazolam PCS system in the ICU population.[237] Beginning with incremental doses of 0.25 mg and a lockout interval of 10 minutes, these patients decreased their anxiety score and morphine use and were amnestic of invasive or painful events. There were no instances of hemodynamic or respiratory compromise and their decreased anxiety was noted by the physicians and nurses. PCS has been successful with a variety of agents in the ambulatory surgical patient[238] and during epidural anesthesia,[239] with greater satisfaction than anesthesiologist-controlled sedation.[239]

CONCLUSIONS

Patient-controlled analgesia (PCA) via programmable infusion pumps has proven effective and is superior to conventional parenteral regimens with fewer side effects than epidural narcotics. Advantages include a flexible strategy with the patient in control, more physiologic administration than other parenteral bolus techniques, decreased nonanalgesic waiting time for drug administration, consistent drug serum levels, decreased side effects compared with conventional administration, and few contraindications. There may be no decrease in total narcotic dose levels with this technique, and patient variability prevents cook book dosage formulae. This technique allows the patient to define the limits of his or her narrow and dynamic therapeutic window. To be successful, PCA requires physicians and nurses to diligently interact with patients to adjust the dosing regimens to the patient's response. These attributes make intravenous patient-controlled analgesia an effective tool in the management of pain following thoracic surgery.

References

1. Roe BB: Are postoperative narcotics necessary. Arch Surg 87:912, 1963
2. Cronin M, Redfern PA, Utting JE: Psychometry and postoperative pain complaints in surgical patients. Br J Anaesth 45:879, 1973
3. Sriwatanakul K, Weis OF, Alloza JL et al: Analysis of narcotic analgesic usage in the treatment of postoperative pain. JAMA 250:926, 1983
4. Weis OF, Sriwatanakul K, Alloza JL et al: Attitudes of patients, house-staff and nurses toward postoperative analgesic care. Anesth Analg 62:70, 1983
5. Marks RM, Sachar EJ: Undertreatment of medical inpatients with narcotic analgesics. Ann Intern Med 78:173, 1973
6. Cohen FL: Post surgical pain relief: Patients' status and nurses' medication choices. Pain 9:265, 1980
7. Parkhouse J, Lambrechts W, Simpson BRJ: The incidence of postoperative pain. Br J Anaesth 33:345, 1961
8. Utting JE, Smith JM: Postoperative analgesia. Anaesthesia 34:320, 1979
9. Editorial: Tight fisted analgesia. Lancet 1:1338, 1976
10. Donald I: At the receiving end. Scot Med J 21:49, 1976
11. Angell M: Editorial: The quality of mercy. N Engl J Med 306:98, 1982
12. Max MB: Improving outcomes of analgesic treatment: Is education enough? Ann Intern Med 113:885, 1990
13. Solecki RS, Shanidar N: A Neanderthal flower burial in Northern Iraq. Science 190:880, 1975
14. Editorial: Postoperative pain. Br Med J 2:517, 1978
15. Benedetti C, Bonica J, Bellucci G: Pathophysiology and therapy of postoperative pain: A review. In Benedetti C, Chapman RC, Moricca G (eds). Advances in Pain Research and Therapy, p. 7. New York, Raven Press, 1984
16. Sechzer PH: Objective measurement of pain. Anesthesiology 29:209, 1968

17. Pflug AE, Bonica JJ: Physiopathology and control of postoperative pain. Arch Surg 112:773, 1977
18. Raj PP: Epidemiology of pain. In Raj PP (ed). Practical Management of Pain, p. 14. Chicago, Yearbook Medical Publishers, 1986
19. Bonica JJ: Foreword. In Paris PM, Stewart RD (eds). Pain Management in Emergency Medicine, p. xii. Norwalk: Appleton and Lange, 1988
20. Merskey H: Classification of chronic pain, descriptions of chronic pain syndromes and definitions of pain terms. Pain suppl 3, 1986
21. Bonica JJ: Importance of the problem. In Arnoff GM (ed). Evaluation and treatment of chronic pain, p. xxxi. Baltimore: Urban and Schwarzenberg, 1985
22. Wall PD: On the relationship of injury to pain. Pain 6:253, 1979
23. Chapman CR, Casey KL, Dubner R et al: Pain measurement: An overview. Pain 22:1, 1985
24. Melzack R: The McGill pain questionnaire. In Melzack R (ed). Pain Measurement and Assessment, p. 41. New York, Raven Press, 1983
25. Bonica JJ: Definitions and taxonomy of pain. In Bonica JJ (ed). The Management of Pain, p. 19. Philadelphia, Lea & Febiger, 1990
26. Charlton JE, Gagliardi G, Klein R et al: Factors affecting pain in burned patients: A preliminary report. Postgrad Med J 59:604, 1983
27. Spence AA, Smith G: Postoperative analgesia and lung function: A comparison of morphine with extradural block. Br J Anaesth 43:144, 1971
28. Meyers JR, Lambeck L, O'Kane H et al: Changes in functional residual capacity of the lung after operation. Arch Surg 110:576, 1975
29. Craig DB: Postoperative recovery of pulmonary function. Anesth Analg 60:46, 1981
30. Jaattela A, Alho A, Avikainen V et al: Plasma catecholamine in severely injured patients: A prospective study of 45 patients with multiple injuries. Br J Surg 62:177, 1975
31. Kehlet H: The stress response to anaesthesia and surgery: Release mechanisms and modifying factors. Clin Anesth 2:315, 1984
32. Gelfand RA, Matthews DE, Bier DM: Role of counterregulatory hormones in the catabolic response to stress. J Clin Invest 74:2238, 1984
33. Kehlet H, Brandt MR, Rem J: Role of neurogenic stimuli in mediating the endocrine-metabolic response to surgery. J Par Ent Nutr 4:152, 1980
34. Cuthlartson DP: The metabolic response to injury and its nutritional implications: Retrospect and prospect. J Par Ent Nutr 3:108, 1979
35. Wilmore DW, Aulick LH: Metabolic changes in burned patients. Surg Clin North Am 58:1173, 1978
36. Christenson P, Brandt MR, Rem J et al: Influence of extradural morphine on the adrenocortical and hyperglycemic response to surgery. Br J Anaesth 54:24, 1982
37. Jorgensen BC, Anderson HB, Engquist A: Influence of epidural morphine on postoperative pain, endocrine metabolic and renal responses to surgery: A controlled study. Acta Anaesthesiol Scand 26:63, 1982
38. Kehet H, Brandt MR, Prange Hansen A et al: Effect of epidural analgesia on metabolic profiles during and after surgery. Br J Surg 66:543, 1979
39. Bromage PR, Shibata HR, Willoughby HW: Influence of prolonged epi-

dural blockade on blood sugar and cortisol responses to operations upon the upper part of the abdomen and thorax. Surg Gynecol Obstet 132:1051, 1971

40. Bevan DR: Modification of the metabolic response to trauma under extradural analgesia. Anaesthesia 26:189, 1971

41. Engquist A, Brandt MR, Fernandes A et al: The blocking effect of epidural analgesia on the adrenocortical and hyperglycemic response to surgery. Acta Anaesthesiol Scand 21:330, 1977

42. Phillips GD, Cousins MJ: Neurological mechanisms of pain and the relationship of pain, anxiety and sleep. In Cousins MJ, Phillips GD (eds). Acute Pain Management, p. 21. New York, Churchill Livingstone, Inc., 1986

43. McKegney FP: The intensive care syndrome: Definition, treatment, and prevention of a new "disease of medical progress." Conn Med 30:633, 1966

44. Keats AS: Postoperative pain: Research and treatment. J Chronic Dis 4:72, 1956

45. Donovan M, Dillon P, McGuire L: Incidence and characteristics of pain in a sample of medical–surgical inpatients. Pain 6:249, 1987

46. Mather LE, Phillips GD: Opioids and adjuvants: Principles of use. In Cousins MJ, Phillips GD (eds). Acute Pain Management, p. 77. New York, Churchill Livingstone, Inc., 1986

47. Porter J, Jick H: Addiction rare in patients treated with narcotics [Letter]. N Engl J Med 302:123, 1980

48. Miller RR: Clinical effects of parenteral narcotics in hospitalized medical patients. J Clin Pharmacol 20:165, 1980

49. Miller RR: Analgesics. In Miller RR, Greenblatt DJ (eds). Drug Effects in Hospitalized Patients, p. 151. New York, John Wiley and Sons, 1976

50. Wolman RL, Luterman A: The continuous infusion of morphine sulfate for analgesia in burn patients: Extending the use of an established technique (abstr). Am Burn Assoc 20:150, 1988

51. Mather LE, Owen H: The scientific basis of patient-controlled analgesia. Anaesth Intensive Care 16:427, 1988

52. Wolman RL, Shapiro JH: Pain management in the critically ill. In Taylor RW, Shoemaker WC (eds). Critical Care: State of the Art, XII, p. 417. Fullerton, CA, The Society of Critical Care Medicine, 1991

53. Stapleton JV, Austin KL, Mather LE: Postoperative pain [Letter]. Br Med J 2:1449, 1978

54. Graves DA, Foster TS, Batenhorst RL, Bennett RL, Baumann TJ: Patient-controlled analgesia. Ann Intern Med 99:360, 1983

55. Vache E: Inadequate treatment of pain in hospitalized patients [Letter]. N Engl J Med 307:55, 1982

56. Twycross RG: Ethical and clinical aspects of pain treatment in cancer patients. Acta Anaesthesiol Scand [Suppl] 26(suppl 74):83, 1982

57. Austin KL, Stapleton JV, Mather LE: Multiple intramuscular injections a major source of variability in analgesic response to meperidine. Pain 8:47, 1980

58. Austin KL, Stapleton JV, Mather LE: Relationship between blood meperidine concentrations and analgesic response: A preliminary report. Anesthesiology 53:460, 1980

59. Bellville JW, Forrest WH Jr, Miller E et al: Influence of age on pain relief from analgesics—A study of postoperative patients. JAMA 217:1835, 1971

60. Tamsen A, Hartvig P, Fagerlund C, Dahlstrom B: Patient-controlled analgesic therapy, Part II: Individual analgesic demand and analgesic plasma concentrations of pethidine in postoperative pain. Clin Pharmacokinet 7:164, 1982

61. Tamsen A, Bondesson U, Dahlstrom B, Hartvig P: Patient-controlled analgesic therapy, Part III: Pharmacokinetics and analgesic plasma concentrations of ketobemidone. Clin Pharmacokinet 7:252, 1982

62. Dahlstrom B, Tamsen A, Paalzow L, Hartvig P: Patient-controlled analgesic therapy, Part IV: Pharmacokinetics and analgesic plasma concentrations of morphine. Clin Pharmacokinet 7:266, 1982

63. Kaiko RF, Wallenstein SL, Rogers AG, Houde RW: Sources of variation in analgesic responses in cancer patients with chronic pain receiving morphine. Pain 15:191, 1983

64. Tamsen A, Sakurda T, Wahlstrom A, Terenius L, Hartvig P: Postoperative demand for analgesics in relation to individual levels on endorphins and substance P in cerebrospinal fluid. Pain 13:171, 1982

65. Tamsen A, Hartvig P, Dahlstrom B, Wahlstrom A, Terenius L: Endorphins and on-demand pain relief. Lancet i:769, 1980

66. Lim AT, Edis G, Kranz H et al: Postoperative pain control: Contributions of psychological factors and transcutaneous electrical nerve stimulation. Pain 17:179, 1983

67. Scott LE, Clum GA, Peoples JB: Preoperative predictors of postoperative pain. Pain 15:283, 1983

68. Egan KJ: What does it mean to a patient to be "in control"? In Ferrante FM, Ostheimer GW, Covino BG (eds). Patient-controlled Analgesia, p. 17. Boston, Blackwell Scientific Publications, Inc., 1990

69. Schorr D, Rodin J: Motivation to control one's environment in individuals with obsessive-compulsive, depressive, and normal personality traits. J Pers Soc Psychol 46:1148, 1984

70. Staub E, Tursky B, Schwartz GE: Self control and predictability: Their effects on reactions to adverse stimulation. J Pers Soc Psychol 18:157, 1971

71. Miller SM: When is a little information a dangerous thing: Coping with stressful events by monitoring vs. blunting. In Levin S, Ursin H (eds). Coping and Health. New York, Plenum, 1980

72. Cromwell RL, Butterfield EC, Brayfield FM, Curry JJ: Acute myocardial infarction: Reaction and recovery. St. Louis: C.V. Mosby, 1977

73. Peck CL: Psychological factors in acute pain management. In Cousins M, Phillips GD (eds). Acute Pain Management, p. 251. New York, Churchill Livingstone, Inc., 1986

74. Chapman CR, Turner JA: Psychological control of acute pain in medical settings. J Pain and Symptom Management 1:9, 1986

75. Thompson SC: Will it hurt less if I can control it: A complex answer to a simple question. Psychol Bull 90:89, 1991

76. Gal R, Lazarus RS: The role of activity in anticipating and confronting stressful situations. J Human Stress 1:4, 1975

77. Ferrante FM, Orav EJ, Rocco AG, Gallo J: A statistical model for pain in patient-controlled analgesia and conventional intramuscular opioid regimens. Anesth Analg 67:457, 1988
78. Edwards DJ, Svensson CK, Visco JP, Lalka D: Clinical pharmacokinetics of pethidine: 1982. Clin Pharmacokinet 7:421, 1982
79. Cockshott WP, Thompson GT, Howlett LJ, Seeley ET: Intramuscular or intralipomatous injections. N Engl J Med 307:356, 1982
80. Catling JA, Pinto DM, Jordon C et al: Respiratory effects of analgesia after cholecystectomy: Comparison of continuous and intermittent papavertetum. Br Med J 2:478, 1980
81. Nayman J: Measurement and control of postoperative pain. Ann Royal Col Surg Engl 61:420, 1979
82. Tamsen A, Hartvig P, Fagerlund C, Dahlstrom B, Bondesson U: Patient-controlled analgesic therapy: Clinical experience. Acta Anaesthesiol Scand 74 (Suppl):157, 1982
83. Keeri-Szanto M: Demand analgesia. In Aldrete JA, Stanley TH (eds). Trends in Intravenous Anesthesia, p. 417. Chicago, Year Book Medical Publishers, 1980
84. Tamsen A: Comparison of patient-controlled analgesia with constant infusion and intermittent intramuscular regimens. In Harmer M, Rosen M, Vickers MD (eds). Patient-controlled analgesia, p. 111. Boston, Blackwell Scientific Publications, 1985
85. Sechzer PH: Patient-controlled analgesia (PCA): A retrospective. Anesthesiology 72:735, 1990
86. Church JJ: Continuous narcotic infusions for relief of postoperative pain. Br Med J 1:977, 1979
87. Bray RJ: Postoperative analgesia provided by morphine infusion in children. Anaesthesia 38:1075, 1983
88. Orr IA, Keenan DJM, Dundee JW: Improved pain relief after thoracotomy: Use of cryoprobe and morphine infusion. Br Med J 283:945, 1981
89. Miser AW, Miser JS, Clark BS: Continuous infusion of morphine sulfate for control of severe pain in children with terminal malignancy. J Pediatr 96:930, 1980
90. Reinburg A, Smolensky MH: Circadian changes of drug disposition in man. Clin Pharmacokinet 7:401, 1982
91. Marshall H, Porteous C, McMillan I et al: Relief of pain by infusion of morphine after operation: Does tolerance develop? Br Med J 291:19, 1985
92. Shealy CN, Maurer D: Transcutaneous nerve stimulation for control of pain. Surg Neurol 2:45, 1974
93. Van der Ark GD, McGrath KA: Transcutaneous electrical stimulation in the treatment of postoperative pain. Am J Surg 130:338, 1975
94. Tyler E, Caldwell C, Ghia JN: Transcutaneous electrical nerve stimulation: An alternative approach to the management of postoperative pain. Anesth Analg 61:449, 1982
95. Cooperman AM, Hall B, Mikalacki K et al: Use of transcutaneous electrical stimulation in control of postoperative pain—Results of a prospective, randomized, controlled study. Am J Surg 133:185, 1977
96. Ali JA, Yaffee CS, Serretti C: The effect of transcutaneous nerve stim-

ulation on postoperative pain and pulmonary function. Surgery 89:507, 1981

97. Pike PM: Transcutaneous electrical stimulation: Its use in management of postoperative pain. Anaesthesia 33:165, 1978

98. Kimball KL, Drews JE, Walker S et al: Use of TENS for pain reduction in burn patients receiving travase. J Burn Care Rehab 8:28, 1987

99. Melzack R, Wall PD: Pain mechanisms: A new theory. Science 150:971, 1965

100. Woolf CJ, Mitchell D, Barrett GD: Antinociceptive effect of peripheral segmental electrical stimulation in the rat. Pain 8:237, 1980

101. Solomon RA, Viernstein MC, Lang DM: Reduction of postoperative pain and narcotic use by transcutaneous electrical nerve stimulation. Surgery 87:142, 1980

102. Deyo RA, Walsh NE, Martin DC et al: A controlled trial of transcutaneous electrical nerve stimulation (TENS) and exercise for low back pain. N Engl J Med 322:1627, 1990

103. Hunter AR: Design and calibration of vapourizer for trichlorethylene anaesthesia. Anaesthesia 4:138, 1949

104. Hall KD: The analysis of small concentrations of trichlorethylene vapor by inferometry. Anesthesiology 14:38, 1953

105. Romangnoli A, Korman D: Methoxyflurane in obstetrical anesthesia and analgesia. Can Anaesth Soc J 9:414, 1962

106. Bodley PO, Mirza V, Spears JR, Spilsbury RA: Obstetrical analgesia with methoxyflurane: A clinical trial. Anaesthesia 21:457, 1966

107. Yakaitis RW, Redding JS: Self-administered methoxyflurane for improved postoperative ventilation. Anesth Analg 49:345, 1970

108. Filkins SA, Cosgrave P, Marvin JA et al: Self administered anesthetic: A method of pain control. J Burn Care Rehab 1:33, 1981

109. Forrest WH, Smethurst PWR, Kienitz ME: Self-administration of intravenous analgesics. Anesthesiology 33:363, 1970

110. Sechzer PH: Studies in pain with the analgesic-demand system. Anesth Analg 50:1, 1971

111. Keeri-Szanto M, Heaman S: Postoperative analgesic demand. Surg Gynecol Obstet 134:647, 1972

112. Keeri-Szanto M: Apparatus for demand analgesia. Can Anaesth Soc J 18:581, 1971

113. Evans JM, MacCarthy J, Rosen M et al: Apparatus for patient-controlled administration of intravenous narcotics during labour. Lancet i:17, 1976

114. Bohr M, Rosen M, Vickers MD: Self-administered nalbuphine, morphine and pethidine: Comparison by intravenous route following cholecystectomy. Anaesthesia 40:529, 1985

115. Chakravaty K, Tucker W, Rosen M et al: Comparison of buprenorphine and pethidine given intravenously on demand to relieve postoperative pain. Br Med J 2:895, 1979

116. Harmer M, Slattery PJ, Rosen M et al: Comparison between buprenorphine and pentazocine given i.v. on demand in the control of postoperative pain. Br J Anaesth 55:21, 1983

117. Slattery PJ, Harmer M, Rosen M et al: Comparison of meptazinol and

pethidine given IV on demand in the management of postoperative pain. Br J Anaesth 53:927, 1981

118. Sprigge JS, Otton PE: Nalbuphine versus meperidine for postoperative analgesia: A double-blind comparison using the patient-controlled analgesic technique. Can Anaesth Soc J 30:517, 1983

119. Hull CJ, Sibbald A: Control of postoperative pain by interactive demand analgesia. Br J Anaesth 53:385, 1981

120. Hull CJ, Sibbald A, Johnson MK: Demand analgesia for postoperative pain. Br J Anaesth 51:570, 1979

121. Tamsen A, Hartvig P, Dahlstrom B, Lindstrom B, Holmdahl MH: Patient-controlled analgesia therapy in the early postoperative period. Acta Anaesth Scand 23:462, 1979

122. Tamsen A, Hartvig P, Fagerlund C et al: Patient-controlled analgesic therapy: Pharmacokinetics of pethidine in the pre- and postoperative periods. Clin Pharmacokinet 7:149, 1982

123. Bennett RL, Baumann T, Batenhorst RL et al: Morphine titration in postoperative laparotomy patients using patient-controlled analgesia. Curr Ther Res 32:45, 1982

124. Bennett RL, Batenhorst RL, Graves D et al: Patient-controlled analgesia: A new concept of postoperative relief. Ann Surg 195:700, 1982

125. Bennett RL, Batenhorst RL, Graves D et al: Variation in postoperative analgesic requirements in the morbidly obese following gastric bypass surgery. Pharmacother 2:43, 1982

126. Graves DA, Batenhorst RL, Bennett RL et al: Morphine requirements using patient-controlled analgesia: Influence of diurnal variation and morbid obesity. Clin Pharm 2:49, 1983

127. Norman J: Terminology used in patient-controlled analgesia. In Harmer M, Rosen M, Vickers MD (eds). Patient-controlled Analgesia, p. 3. Boston, Blackwell Scientific Publications, Inc., 1985

128. White PF: Patient-controlled analgesia: Delivery systems. In Ferrante FM, Ostheimer GW, Covino BG (eds). Patient-controlled Analgesia, p. 70. Boston, Blackwell Scientific Publications, Inc., 1990

129. Hull CJ, McCarthy JP, Tamsen A, Bennett RL, White PF et al: Apparatus. In Harmer M, Rosen M, Vickers MD (eds). Patient-controlled Analgesia, p. 83. Boston, Blackwell Scientific Publications, Inc., 1985

130. White PF: Patient-controlled analgesia: An update on its use in the treatment of postoperative pain. Anesthesiology Clin North Am 7:63, 1989

131. White PF: Patient-controlled analgesia: A new approach to the management of postoperative pain. Semin Anesth 4:255, 1985

132. White PF: Patient-controlled analgesia. Problems in Anesthesia 2:339, 1988

133. Ferrante FM, Ostheimer GW, Covino BG (eds). Patient-controlled analgesia. Boston, Blackwell Scientific Publications, Inc., 1990

134. Harmer M, Rosen M, Vickers MD (eds). Patient-controlled analgesia. Boston, Blackwell Scientific Publications, Inc., 1985

135. Finley RJ, Keeri-Szanto M, Boyd D: New analgesic agents and techniques shorten postoperative hospital stay. Pain 2:S397, 1984

136. Bollish SJ, Collins CL, Kirking DM, Bartlett RH: Efficacy of patient-

controlled versus conventional analgesia for postoperative pain. Clin Pharm 4:48, 1985

137. Rosenberg PH, Heino A, Scheinin B: Comparison of intramuscular analgesia, intercostal block, epidural morphine, and on-demand-i.v.-fentanyl in the control of pain after upper abdominal surgery. Acta Anaesthesiol Scand 28:603, 1984

138. Slattery PJ, Harmer M, Rosen M, Vickers MD: An open comparison between routine and self-administered postoperative pain relief. Ann Royal Coll Surg Engl 65:18, 1983

139. Eisenach JC, Grice SC, Dewan DM: Patient-controlled analgesia following Cesarean section: A comparison with epidural and intramuscular narcotics. Anesthesiology 68:444, 1988

140. Wasylak TJ, Abbott FV, English MJ, Jeans ME: Reduction of postoperative morbidity following patient-controlled morphine. Can J Anaesth 37:726, 1990

141. Editorial: Patient-controlled analgesia. Lancet 1:289, 1980

142. Atwell JR, Flanigan RC, Bennett RL et al: The efficacy of patient-controlled analgesia in patients recovering from flank incisions. J Urol 132:701, 1984

143. Bennett RL, Griffen WO: Effect of patient-controlled analgesia on nocturnal sleep and spontaneous activity following laparotomy (abstr). Anesthesiology 61:A205, 1984

144. Bennett RL, Batenhorst RL, Bivens BA et al: Drug use pattern in patient-controlled analgesia (abstr). Anesthesiology 57:A210, 1982

145. Keeri-Szanto M: Drugs or drums: What relieves postoperative pain? Pain 6:217, 1979

146. Ellis R, Haines D, Shah R et al: Pain relief after abdominal surgery: Comparison of i.m. morphine, sublingual buprenorphine, and self-administered i.v. pethidine. Br J Anaesth 54:421, 1982

147. Welchew EA: On-demand analgesia: A double blind comparison of on-demand intravenous fentanyl with regular intramuscular morphine. Anaesthesia 38:19, 1983

148. Dahl JB, Daugaard JJ, Larsen HV, Mourridsen P et al: Patient-controlled analgesia: A controlled trial. Acta Anaesthesiol Scand 31:744, 1987

149. Robinson SL, Fell D: Nausea and vomiting with the use of a patient-controlled analgesia system. Anaesthesia 46:580, 1991

150. Harrison DM, Sinatra R, Moorgese L, Chung JH: Epidural narcotic and patient-controlled analgesia for post-cesearean section pain relief. Anesthesiology 68:454, 1988

151. Bolden M, Patel R, de la Vega S, McKenzie R: Patient-controlled analgesic following elective cesarean delivery. SOAP, 1985

152. White PF: Use of patient-controlled analgesia for management of acute pain. JAMA 259:243, 1988

153. Bennett RL, Batenhorst RL, Foster TS, Griffen WO, Wright BD: Postoperative pulmonary function with patient-controlled analgesia (abstr). Anesth Analg 61:171, 1982

154. Schechter NL, Berrien FB, Katz SM: The use of patient-controlled analgesia in adolescents with sickle cell pain crisis: A preliminary report. J Pain and Symptom Management 3:109, 1988

155. Vickers MD: Clinical trials of analgesic drugs. In Harmer M, Rosen M, Vickers MD (eds). Patient-controlled Analgesia, p. 42. Boston, Blackwell Scientific Publications, Inc., 1985

156. Lange MP, Dahn MS, Jacobs LA: Patient-controlled analgesia versus intermittent analgesia dosing. Heart & Lung 17:495, 1988

157. Wang CS, Chou YP, Hou CC, Li CY et al: Efficiency of patient-controlled analgesia versus conventional analgesia in patients after thoracotomy. Ma Tsui Hsueh Tsa Chi 29:604, 1991

158. Wolman RL, Lasecki MH, Alexander LA, Luterman A: Clinical trial of patient controlled analgesia in burn patients (abstr). Am Burn Assoc 19:166, 1987

159. White DC, Pearce DJ, Norman J: Postoperative analgesia: A comparison of intravenous on-demand fentanyl with epidural bupivacaine. Br Med J 2:166, 1979

160. Cohen SE, Suback LL, Brose WG, Halpern J: Anesthesia after cesarean delivery: Patient evaluations and costs of five opioid techniques. Reg Anesth 16:141, 1991

161. Weller RS, Rosenblum M, Conard P, Gross JB: "Smoother" pain control with epidural vs. patient-controlled i.v. morphine following joint replacement surgery (abstr). Anesthesiology 73:A823, 1990

162. Purves PG, Sperring SJ, Dykes V, Stanley TD: Improved postoperative analgesia: Epidural vs patient controlled intravenous morphine (abstr). Anesth Analg 66:S143, 1987

163. Weller RS, Rosenblum M, Conard P, Gross JB: Comparison of epidural and patient-controlled intravenous morphine following joint replacement surgery. Can J Anaesth 38:582, 1991

164. Rockemann MG, Seeling W, Bothner U, Eifert B, Zeininger A: Postoperative outcome after abdominal surgery: Patient controlled analgesia versus epidural analgesia with morphine or bupivacaine/morphine (abstr). Anesthesiology 75:A1088, 1991

165. Bellamy CD, McDonnell FJ, Colclough GW: Postoperative epidural pain management results in shorter hospital stay than IV PCA morphine: A comparison in anterior cruciate ligament repair (abstr). Anesthesiology 71:A686, 1989

166. Norris EJ, Parker S, Breslow MJ et al: The endocrine response to surgical stress: A comparison of epidural anesthesia/analgesia vs. general anesthesia/patient-controlled analgesia (abstr). Anesthesiology 75: A696, 1991

167. Benzon HT, Wong HY, Velavic A, Locicero J: Double-blind comparison of epidural fentanyl and PCA morphine in post-thoracotomy pain (abstr). Anesthesiology 75:A712, 1991

168. Wong HY, Benzon HT, LoCicerl J: Use of placebo PCA by patients receiving epidural fentanyl analgesia (abstr). Anesth Analg 74:S356, 1992

169. Gourlay GK, Kowalski SR, Plummer JL, Cousins MJ, Armstrong PJ: Fentanyl blood concentration—Analgesic response relationship in the treatment of postoperative pain. Anesth Analg 67:329, 1988

170. Lehmann KA, Gerhard A, Horrichs-Haermeyer G, Grond S, Zech D: Postoperative patient-controlled analgesia with sufentanil: Analgesic efficacy and minimum effective concentrations. Acta Anaesthesiol Scand 35:221, 1991

171. Lehmann KA, Gordes B, Hoeckle W: Postoperative on-demand analgesia with morphine. Anaesthetist 34:494, 1985
172. Welchew EA, Hosking J: Patient-controlled postoperative analgesia with alfentanil: Adaptive, on-demand intravenous alfentanil or pethidine compared double-blind for postoperative pain. Anaesthesia 40:1172, 1985
173. Lehmann KA, Grond S, Freier J, Zech D: Postoperative pain management and respiratory depression after thoracotomy: A comparison of intramuscular piritramide and intravenous patient-controlled analgesia using fentanyl or buprenorphine. J Clin Anesth 3:194, 1991
174. Smith CV, Rayburn WF, Karaiskakis PT, Morton RD, Norvell MJ: Comparison of patient-controlled analgesia and epidural morphine for postcesarean pain and recovery. J Reprod Med 36:430, 1991
175. Vanhoorebeeck P, Vertommen JD, Van Aken H, Vandermeersch E: Vital capacity after thoracotomy: Continuous epidural fentanyl vs. intravenous patient-controlled analgesia (abstr). Anesthesiology 75:A116, 1991
176. McKenzie R, Rudy T, Tantisira B: Comparison of PCA alone and PCA with continuous infusion on pain relief and quality of sleep (abstr). Anesthesiology 73:A787, 1990
177. Sinatra R, Chung KS, Silverman DG et al: An evaluation of morphine and oxymorphone administered via patient-controlled analgesia (PCA) or PCA plus basal infusion in postcesarean-delivery patients. Anesthesiology 71:502, 1989
178. Berde CB, Yee JD, Lehn BM, Moore LJ, Sethna NF: Patient-controlled analgesia in children and adolescents: A comparison with intramuscular morphine (abstr). Anesthesiology 73:A1102, 1990
179. Silverman DG, Preble LM, Paige D, O'Connor TZ, Brull SJ: Basal infusion as supplement to PCA in orthopedic patients (abstr). Anesth Analg 72:S256, 1990
180. Hansen LA, Noyes MA, Lehman ME: Evaluation of patient-controlled analgesia (PCA) versus PCA plus continuous infusion in postoperative cancer patients. J Pain and Symptom Management 6:4, 1991
181. Parker RK, Holtman B, White PF: Patient-controlled analgesia. Does concurrent opioid infusion improve pain management after surgery? JAMA 266:1947, 1991
182. Owen H, Currie JC, Plummer JL: Variation in the blood concentration/analgesic response relationship during patient-controlled analgesia with alfentanil. Anaesth Intensive Care 19:555, 1991
183. Vinik HR, Hammonds W, Lett A et al: Patient-controlled analgesia (PCA) combined with continuous infusion (CI) (abstr). Anesth Analg 70:S418, 1990
184. Owen H, Szekely SM, Plummer JL et al: Variables of patient-controlled analgesia 2: Concurrent infusion. Anaesthesia 44:11, 1989
185. Sinatra RS, Lodge K, Sibert K et al: A comparison of morphine, meperidine, and oxymorphone as utilized in patient-controlled analgesia following cesarean section. Anesthesiology 70:585, 1989
186. Ginsberg B, Gil KM, Muir M, Sykes D: PCA: Correlation between narcotic use, pain and psychological parameters (abstr). Anesthesiology 71:A687, 1989

187. Lehmann KA, Tenbuhs B, Hoeckle W: Patient controlled analgesia with piritramide for the treatment of postoperative pain. Acta Anaesthesiol Belg 37:247, 1986
188. Lehmann KA, Gordes B: Postoperative on-demand analgesia with buprenorphine. Anaesthesist 37:65, 1988
189. Parker RK, Perry F, Holtmann B, White PF: Demographic factors influencing the PCA morphine requirement (abstr). Anesthesiology 73: A818, 1990
190. Ginsberg B, Cohen NA, Ossey KD, Glass PSA: The use of PCA to assess the influence of demographic factors on analgesic requirements (abstr). Anesthesiology 71:A688, 1989
191. Monk TG, Parker RK, White PF: Use of PCA in geriatric patients—Effects of aging on the postoperative analgesic requirement (abstr). Anesth Analg 70:S272, 1990
192. Berkowitz BA, Ngai SH, Yang JC, Hempstead J, Spector S: The disposition of morphine in surgical patients. Clin Pharmacol Ther 17:629, 1975
193. Greenblatt DJ, Sellers EM, Shader RI: Drug disposition in old age. N Engl J Med 306:1081, 1982
194. Magnani BJ, Johnson LR, Ferrante FM: Modifiers of patient-controlled analgesia efficacy. II. Chronic pain. Pain 39:23, 1989
195. Ready LB, Oden R, Chadwick HS et al: Development of an anesthesiology-based postoperative pain management service. Anesthesiology 68:100, 1988
196. Stacey BR, Brody MC, Burke DF: Patients with a substance abuse history can effectively use PCA (abstr). Anesthesiology 73:A760, 1990
197. Beyer JE, DeGood DE, Ashley LC et al: Patterns of postoperative analgesic use with adults and children following cardiac surgery. Pain 17:71, 1983
198. Mather L, Mackie J: The incidence of postoperative pain in children. Pain 15:271, 1983
199. Tyler DC: Respiratory effects of pain in a child after thoracotomy. Anesthesiology 70:873, 1989
200. Haberken CM, Tyler DC, Krane EJ: Postoperative pain management in children. Mt Sinai J Med 58:247, 1991
201. Rodgers BM, Webb CJ, Stergios C, Newman BM: Patient-controlled analgesia in pediatric surgery. J Pediatr Surg 23:259, 1988
202. Browne RE, Broadman LM: Patient-controlled analgesia (PCA) for postoperative pain control in adolescents (abstr). Anesth Analg 66:S22, 1987
203. Broadman LM: Patient-controlled analgesia in children and adolescents. In: Ferrante FM, Ostheimer GW, Covino BG (eds). Patient-controlled Analgesia, p. 129. Boston, Blackwell Scientific Publications, Inc., 1990
204. Broadman L, Vaughan M, Rice L, Randolph J: Patient controlled analgesia provides more effective postoperative pain control following pectus excavatum repair in children than does conventional narcotic therapy (abstr). Anesthesiology 71:A1045, 1989
205. Broadman LM, Brown RE, Rice LJ, Higgins T, Vaughan M: Patient controlled analgesia in children and adolescents: A report of postoperative

pain management in 150 patients (abstr). Anesthesiology 71:A1171, 1989

206. Lawrie SC, Forbes DW, Akhtar TM, Morton NS: Patient-controlled analgesia in children. Anaesthesia 45:1074, 1990

207. Mowbray MJ, Gaukroger PB: Long-term patient-controlled analgesia in children. Anaesthesia 45:941, 1990

208. Berde CB, Lehn BM, Yee JD, Sethna NF, Russo D: Patient-controlled analgesia in children and adolescents: A randomized, prospective comparison with intramuscular administration of morphine for postoperative analgesia. J Pediatr 118:460, 1991

209. White PF: Mishaps with patient-controlled analgesia. Anesthesiology 66:81, 1987

210. Wakerlin G, Larson CP: Spouse-controlled analgesia [Letter]. Anesth Analg 70:119, 1990

211. VanDercar DH, Martinez AP, De Lisser EA: Sleep apnea syndromes: A potential contraindication for patient-controlled analgesia. Anesthesiology 74:623, 1991

212. McKenzie R: Patient-controlled analgesia (PCA) [Letter]. Anesthesiology 69:1027, 1988

213. Grey TC, Sweeny ES: Patient-controlled analgesia. JAMA 259:2240, 1988

214. Riley RH, Coppinger GC: PCA activation by reinsertion of a power cord [Letter]. Anaesth Intensive Care 19:132, 1991

215. Kluger MT, Owen H: Antireflux valves in patient-controlled analgesia. Anaesthesia 45:1057, 1990

216. Stevens DS, Cohen RI, Kanzaria RV, Dunn WT Jr: Air in the syringe: Patient-controlled analgesia machine tampering. Anesthesiology 75:697, 1991

217. Ready LB: The economics of patient-controlled analgesia. In Ferrante FM, Ostheimer GW, Covino BG (eds). Patient-controlled Analgesia, p. 191. Boston, Blackwell Scientific Publications, Inc., 1990

218. Rao MK, Balcueva EP, Thiem C, Bommarito AA: Evaluation of demand analgesia in a community hospital. Resident and Staff Physician 32:26, 1986

219. Chrubasik J, Wiemers D: Continuous-plus-on-demand epidural infusion of morphine for postoperative pain relief by means of a small, externally worn infusion device. Anesthesiology 62:263, 1985

220. Parker RK, Baron M, Helfer DL, Berberich N, White PF: Epidural PCA: Effect of a continuous (basal) infusion on the postoperative opioid requirement (abstr). Anesth Analg 70:S296, 1990

221. Boudreault D, Brasseur L, Samii K, Lemoing JP: Comparison of continuous epidural bupivacaine infusion plus either continuous epidural infusion or patient-controlled epidural injection of fentanyl for postoperative analgesia. Anesth Analg 73:132, 1991

222. Estok PM, Glass PSA, Goldberg JS, Freiberger JJ, Sladen RN: Use of patient-controlled analgesia to compare intravenous to epidural administration of fentanyl in the postoperative patient (abstr). Anesthesiology 67:A230, 1987

223. Hongnat M, Bellenfant F, Levy R, Alfonsi P, Chauvin M: Epidural versus intravenous alfentanil by PCA in postoperative patients (abstr). Anesthesiology 75:A754, 1991

224. Sjostrom S, Hartvig D, Tamsen A: Patient-controlled analgesia with extradural morphine or pethidine. Br J Anaesth 60:358, 1988

225. Welchew EA, Breen DP: Patient-controlled on-demand epidural fentanyl. A comparison of patient-controlled on-demand fentanyl delivered epidurally or intravenously. Anaesthesia 46:438, 1991

226. Bustamante J, Sawaki Y, White PF: Comparison of IV-PCA vs. Epidural-PCA following major vascular surgery (abstr). Anesth Analg 74:S39, 1992

227. Prados W, Renfroe D: Route of PCA affects incidence of urinary retention following orthopedic surgery (abstr). Anesthesiology 75:A751, 1991

228. Walmsley PNH, Colclough GW, Mazloomdoost M, McDonnell FJ: Epidural PCA/infusion for post-nephrectomy pain: Shorter hospitalization (abstr). Anesthesiology 71:A684, 1989

229. Urquhart ML, Klapp K, White P: Patient-controlled analgesia: A comparison of intravenous versus subcutaneous hydromorphone. Anesthesiology 69:428, 1988

230. Taylor E, White PF, Urquhart ML: Postoperative analgesia: SQ-PCA vs. IV-PCA (abstr). Anesthesiology 71:A685, 1989

231. Bruera E: Ambulatory infusion devices in the continuing care of patients with advanced diseases. J Pain and Symptom Management 5:287, 1990

232. Bruera E, MacMillan K, Hanson J, MacDonald RN: The Edmonton injector: A simple device for patient-controlled subcutaneous analgesia. Pain 44:167, 1991

233. Shah MV, Jones DI, Rosen M: "Patient demand" postoperative analgesia with buprenorphine: Comparison between sublingual and i.m. administration. Br J Anaesth 58:508, 1986

234. Lu SL, Wang JL, Wenz RZ, Wang QA: Clinical application of a patient-controlled apparatus for ventricular administration of morphine in intractable pain: Report of 28 cases. Neurosurgery 29:73, 1991

235. Strain JJ: Psychological reactions to acute medical illness and critical care. Crit Care Med 6:39, 1978

236. Gowan NJ: The perceptual world of the intensive care unit: An overview of some of the environmental considerations in the helping relationship. Heart & Lung 8:340, 1979

237. Loper KA, Ready A, Ready LB, Brody M: Patient-controlled anxiolysis with midazolam. Anesth Analg 67:1118, 1988

238. Ghouri AF, Tekonda R, Taylor E, White PF: Patient controlled sedation: A comparison of three techniques during local anesthesia (abstr). Anesth Analg 74:S110, 1992

239. Park WY, Watkins PA: Patient-controlled sedation during epidural analgesia. Anesth Analg 72:304, 1991

Pain Management in Cardiothoracic Surgery, edited by Gravlee and Rauck. J. B. Lippincott Company, Philadelphia © 1993.

P. Prithvi Raj
James E. Brannon

4 | Analgesic Considerations for the Median Sternotomy

Median sternotomy is performed for a variety of surgical procedures, both cardiac and noncardiac. Sternotomy provides optimal exposure for such noncardiac procedures as excision of retrosternal thyroid tissue, thymectomy, and excision and biopsy of anterior mediastinal masses. Cardiac procedures requiring median sternotomy include coronary artery bypass grafting, valve replacement and repair, repair of ascending aortic arch aneurysms, and repair of a variety of congenital cardiac defects.

Analgesia for acute poststernotomy pain can be provided by any of a number of available modalities. The clinician must consider many important parameters in making his or her prescription for pain relief. One must consider the disease for which the initial procedure was performed as well as other concurrent conditions such as obstructive lung disease, hypertension, diabetes mellitus, renal and hepatic dysfunction, and myasthenia gravis. Another important factor is the need for anticoagulation associated with some procedures; particularly those that require cardiopulmonary bypass (Vide infra).

PAIN MECHANISMS

The pain syndromes that develop poststernotomy are multiple in nature. They can be classified according to the origin of pain in specific tissues of visceral, musculoskeletal, neurogenic, and dermal origin. They can start as *acute pain*, which may persist and develop into *chronic pain* syndromes. Adequate management of pain during the acute phase may prevent later chronic pain syndromes.

Visceral Pain

Heart

The visceral pain from the heart is transmitted to the central nervous system either via the vagus nerve (parasympathetic) or via the cervical sympathetic (middle and inferior cervical nerves) or the upper five thoracic sympathetic ganglia (thoracic cardiac nerves; Fig. 4–1). Most cardiogenic pain is secondary to ischemia. Whether ischemia is due to coronary artery vasospasm, coronary atherosclerosis, or acute coronary artery insufficiency, the symptoms are usually similar, that is, substernal or epigastric crushing pain, a feeling of tightness, constriction, and heaviness that may become progressively more severe or intense. The pain frequently radiates to the left sternal border, left shoulder, arm, and neck, and there may be an accompanying feeling of impending doom. Acute infectious processes such as endocarditis and myocarditis also produce symptoms of pleuritic substernal or epigastric pain that may be lancinating or paroxysmal, or become continuous and more severe.

Burch and Giles have described a syndrome called cardiac causalgia, which follows the onset of angina pectoris.[1] It is characterized by constant burning and chronic substernal chest discomfort with hyperesthesia of the sternum and the chest wall. Other visceral pains originating from the esophagus, lungs, and ascending arch of the aorta need to be recognized. Their description is not provided in this chapter and is available in other standard textbooks.

Musculoskeletal Pain

Thoracic musculoskeletal pain is a common complaint after sternotomy. It is related to surgical trauma, postsurgical changes, and their sequelae. The site of the pain may involve the vertebrae, the thorax, and the soft tissues surrounding it (Fig. 4–2).

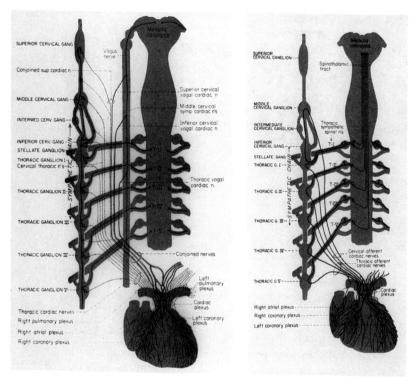

FIGURE 4–1. The autonomic nerve supply to the heart. *Left*, Efferent; *Right*, Afferent nerve supply. *(From Bonica JJ, ed: Sympathetic nerve blocks for pain diagnosis and therapy, Vol. 1. New York, Winthrop Breon, 1984)*

Myofascial Pain

Perhaps the most common persistent pain following thoracic surgery is that emanating from myofascial structures (i.e., muscle, bone, tendon, ligament, and other soft tissues of mesodermal origin). Thoracic fascitis following thoracotomy is common, yet by far the most frequent source of myofascial pain is muscle.

Myofascial pain following sternotomy can involve the anterior and posterior chest wall and the shoulder girdle. The pectoral and serratus anterior muscles are the frequent cause of anterior chest pain, whereas longissimus thoracis and iliocostalis muscles are commonly tender due to myofascial pain. If the shoulder girdle is involved then one might find trapezius, levator scapulae, rhomboid, and supraspinatus muscles painful to touch and in spasm.

The precise mechanism of trigger point generation and perpetuation on muscle following trauma is not known. Simons and Travell[2]

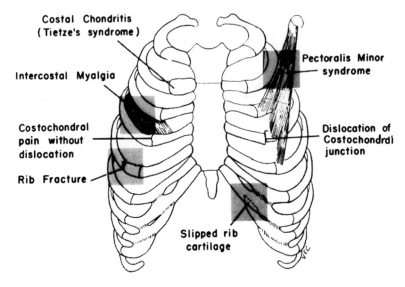

Costal Chondritis (Tietze's syndrome)

Intercostal Myalgia

Pectoralis Minor syndrome

Costochondral pain without dislocation

Dislocation of Costochondral junction

Rib Fracture

Slipped rib cartilage

FIGURE 4–2.   Various causes of thoracic wall pain (anterior).

have hypothesized that transient overload of a muscle may cause damage to the sarcoplasmic reticulum. Stored calcium ions would then be released into the area of injury, and in the presence of adenosine triphosphate (ATP) might activate the actin–myosin contractile mechanism focally in the absence of action potentials. A palpable band of electrically silent muscle would result. Inasmuch as the sarcoplasmic reticulum has been disrupted, calcium reuptake would be limited, and unabated focal contractile activity would persist. High levels of metabolic activity, demonstrated by ATP depletion,[3] produce the "hot spots" seen on infrared thermography. Further, as ATP is required for the Ca-pump to retrieve calcium into the sarcoplasmic reticulum, depletion of ATP further enhances the calcium availability and thus perpetuates contractile activity. Accumulation of metabolic byproducts results in local acidosis, which sensitizes adjacent nociceptors. Increased vascular permeability,[4] local vasoconstriction,[5] and reduced tissue oxygenation[6] also contribute to the elaboration of algesic substances previously described, which sensitize nociceptors.

Costochondritis (Tietze's Syndrome)

True Tietze's Syndrome is most frequently unilateral, involving the second and third costal cartilages (Fig. 4–2).[7–9] The pain is described as mild to moderate over the anterior chest wall and, if severe enough, the patient may confuse the pain with a myocardial infarction. Differential diagnosis includes underlying malignancy and sepsis. Tietze's Syndrome, which is often a diagnosis of exclusion, occurs in all age groups (including children) but is most frequently found in people under the age of 40. Bulbous swellings that may persist for several months and point tenderness over the costochondral junction(s) are characteristic of Tietze's Syndrome. Exacerbations and remissions of the pain can remain localized or radiate to the arm and shoulder.

Additional costochondral pain can arise from trauma to the sternum and ribs, and separation of the ribs, cartilage, and sternum as in median sternotomy. Costochondral arthritis, osteoporosis, infection, trauma, and/or delayed healing following thoracic surgery can challenge therapeutic interventions.

Vertebrae

Painful disorders of the *thoracic vertebrae* may include preexisting osteoporosis, compression fractures, thoracic facet syndrome, ankylosing spondylitis, postural abnormalities (scoliosis), and injuries involving forced or violent flexion or extension movement of the spine. Compression fractures of the thoracic vertebrae due to trauma, osteoporosis secondary to aging or corticosteroid use, and degenerative changes are frequently encountered. The patients complain of localized pain to the back and often of encircling pain following the distribution of the intercostal nerves, aggravated by twisting motions, coughing or postural changes. In the acute setting fractured vertebrae and ribs produce severe, constricting pain of the thorax, which may inhibit respiration. The pain is generally accompanied by severe muscle spasm of the intercostal and paraspinous muscles, inhibiting the patient from obtaining adequate sleep or movement.[10]

Neurogenic Pain

Intercostal Neuralgia

Partial nerve injuries resulting from mechanical trauma sometimes result in an irritative state associated with neuritis. Pain is burning, lancinating, worse at night, and aggravated by stretching the affected nerve. Other irritative phenomena, such as fascicular muscle twitching or spasm, hyperesthesia, paresthesia, or dysesthesia, may be present. Vasomotor or sudomotor changes are usually not seen in the absence of significant sympathetically mediated pain. Intercostal neuralgia following thoracotomy or chest-wall injury is particularly common.

Neuroma

Following complete disruption of a peripheral nerve, the severed ends of the axons continue to grow in an apparent effort to reunite. Anatomical disruption often precludes proper realignment of each proximal axon with its corresponding distal component, which may result in dysesthesia. Abnormal afferent impulses emanating from the dorsal root ganglion following nerve injury also contribute to production of abnormal sensation.[11] In addition, in trauma, or in the case of amputation of a body part, the cut ends of the neurons search in vain for the missing nerve trunk and eventually may curl around themselves in whorl-like fashion or become embedded in scar or other soft tissue. These bulbous collections of nonmyelinated neurons are called *neuromas.*

Neuromas do not behave as normal sensory receptors but instead, when stimulated, often generate an exaggerated response with sharp lancinating pain in the distribution of the affected nerve. Neuromas can be quite labile, causing spontaneous discharge, especially when large and tender.

Scars

In the thoracic region, one can encounter noxious input from cutaneous receptors of a mild-to-severe degree secondary to scar tissue or nerve entrapment. The pain is described as dull and aching, with frequent bouts of sharp, shooting pain associated with particular movement. Local pain can be aggravated by direct pressure on the scar itself, which may then radiate to areas closely associated with the scar tissue or more remote. The patients will complain of exquisite tenderness over the affected area of the scar.

QUALITY OF ACUTE-PAIN MANAGEMENT IN THE PREVENTION OF CHRONIC PAIN

There continues to be increasing evidence that the quality of acute-pain management is an important factor in the subsequent development or prevention of chronic pain.[12,13] Melzack et al.[14] reported that patients with persistent postsurgical pain tended to be older individuals in whom lower doses of analgesics were initially prescribed, resulting in ineffective analgesia in the early postoperative days. Pain persisted for a longer period in these individuals than in individuals in whom early analgesic therapy was effective.

Similarly, anecdotal observations of pretraumatic prophylaxis for pain followed by prolonged analgesia abound. For example, frequently a single dose of subarachnoid morphine administered preoperatively[15] seems to reduce subsequent analgesic requirements during the entire hospital stay of patients undergoing major abdominal and thoracic procedures. Additional controlled studies are obviously needed, but clearly early effective analgesia must be altering typical posttraumatic events. A "critical time interval" has been advanced by Cousins.[16] Effective acute-pain management provided within this interval prevents delayed pain sequelae. Other studies previously mentioned contribute to this impression.[12,13]

The plasticity of the central nervous system permits unmasking of previously unused pain pathways following trauma.[17,18] Some of these changes may be signaled by alterations in substance P and other peptide transport within C fibers. These alterations confuse both diagnosis and treatment in chronic posttraumatic pain.

Algesic substances elaborated in response to trauma (e.g., potassium, serotonin, bradykinin, and histamine) directly activate peripheral pain receptors.[19,20] Other substances such as prostaglandin, substance P, and leukotrienes may play a role in sensitizing primary afferents following trauma.[20,21] One might speculate that this action may also provide a basis for some of the alterations in pain pathways seen in chronic pain states. Early analgesia and primary afferent blockade may in some way alter this chain of events.

Psychological Factors

Psychological factors play an important role in the behavior and adjustment to acute and chronic pain. It may also play a role in the eventual evolution of acute pain into chronic-pain states. Anxiety states, depression, organic brain dysfunction, and posttraumatic stress syndrome can all lead to the expression of pain seemingly out of proportion to what would be typically expected based strictly on the extant physical damage.[22,23] The afferent neural traffic, however, clearly can be altered by psychological factors.[24] Human volunteers have been taught to control the amount of afferent activity as measured by sensatosensory evoked potentials.[25] In other studies, primates have been conditioned so that discharge of pain-transmitting neurons has been observed in anticipation of a noxious stimulus.[26] Perhaps psychological factors may not only alter the outward expression of pain but may also actually increase the afferent barrage following a given traumatic insult.

Early identification of warning signs in the acute (0 to 2 months) and subacute (2 to 6 months) pain stages facilitates aggressive intervention and thus aids in the prevention of chronic-pain states.[22] Denial, anxiety, depression, irritability, family problems, sleep disorders, increasing narcotic use, or dependence on alcohol or tranquilizers are frequent indicators[22] and should be actively searched for in trauma victims.

RESPIRATORY PHYSIOLOGY OF THE MEDIAN STERNOTOMY

There appears to be a consensus that median sternotomy incisions are less painful than lateral thoracotomy incisions, although it would be difficult to perform a controlled study examining this issue. No studies were found that randomly assigned patients undergoing pulmonary resections to median sternotomy or to lateral thoracotomy incisions. Cooper et al. reported nine patients in whom median sternotomy was selected over lateral thoracotomy in order to provide surgical access to both lungs through a single incision.[27] All but one of these patients recovered uneventfully. Had these authors not selected the sternotomy approach, their patients would have required either simultaneous or sequential bilateral thoracotomies, either of which would have almost certainly increased morbidity if not mortality. Cooper et al. also compared vital capacity and peak expiratory flow in 28 patients undergoing either median sternotomy for coronary artery bypass or left lateral thoracotomy for repair of hiatal hernia.[27] At 2 days postoperatively, both vital capacity and peak flow were 40% to 50% of the preoperative values. Although none of the values returned to the preoperative baseline levels by 7 days postoperatively, the median sternotomy group had significantly higher vital capacity and peak flow at 4 and 7 days postoperatively. This was believed to result from less intense pain in that group. Two earlier studies comparing median sternotomy to lateral thoracotomy found little or no difference in postoperative lung function between the two incisions, but one of those studies did not examine postoperative pulmonary function until 4 or more months after surgery.[28,29] Howatt et al. examined the early postoperative time course of pulmonary functional impairment in median sternotomy patients, and found impairment similar to that previously found by others after lateral thoracotomy (i.e., vital capacity 15%–40% of the preoperative values at 1 day postoperatively).[30] Peters et al. found that total pulmonary compliance returned toward normal slightly more quickly after median sternotomy than after lateral thoracotomy, reaching approximately 90% of the preoperative level 7 days after sternotomy while remaining at approximately 70% of the preoperative compliance after lateral thoracotomy.[29] Possibly as a result of those early studies, two subsequent studies combined median sternotomy and lateral thoracotomy into a single category when evaluating the effects of different surgical sites on postoperative pulmonary function and morbidity.[31,32] The rather limited comparative pulmonary physiologic data available thus suggest that, at least for the first 48 hours postoperatively, median sternotomy impairs pulmonary function as much as lateral thoracotomy. This suggests the possibility that creative approaches to early postoperative analgesia might benefit patients undergoing median sternotomy.

MANAGEMENT

Postoperative Pain

An important goal in postsurgical pain management is the early restoration of function. Cellular function depends on blood flow for delivery of nutrients to the tissues. Vasoconstriction, whether secondary to pain or direct vascular injury resulting from trauma or surgical manipulation, interferes with nutrient supply. *Sympathetic blockade* can be used to decrease vascular resistance and improve skin and vascular graft flow, while decreasing pain-mediated vasoconstriction.[33] Regional block for relief of pain can permit improved mobilization on the injured part.[34-35] Early mobilization helps to preserve normal myofascial and gastrointestinal function. Improved nutrient supply, as measured by gastric emptying time, is significantly better with epidural analgesia than with systemic narcotic administration.[37]

A second goal is the modulation of both early and delayed sequelae of pain and injury. Reduced postoperative morbidity has been associated with the use of epidural analgesia in high-risk surgical patients.[38,39] Myofascial pain syndromes resulting from injury to musculoskeletal structures and disuse might well be minimized with early ambulation and mobilization of injured regions.

Modalities of Acute Pain Relief

Systemic Analgesia

Narcotic Analgesics

The mainstay of the analgesic armamentarium for the poststernotomy patient continues to be narcotic analgesics. The exact choice of agent is probably less important than its mode of administration. The intramuscular (IM) route is not suitable for the patient with poor tissue perfusion; intravenous (IV) administration is then the route of choice. IV doses of up to 10 mg of morphine are administered. Small doses are given every 10 minutes until analgesia is adequate.[40] The duration of action of the drug is not critical because additional doses can be given as required. The IV route gives immediate access to the circulation and therefore allows rapid onset of drug action. Rapid distribution and elimination of IV drugs may, however, produce a shorter effect than what is seen following intramuscular injection. Further, short-acting, lipid-soluble narcotics such as fentanyl, alfentanil, or sufentanil are often used to facilitate rapid titration of clinical effect.

The use of a continuous IV infusion makes short-acting narcotic administration practical.[41] The infusion rate can be altered to rapidly produce the desired change in plasma level or clinical effect. This can be achieved with either a conventional IV set and an infusion pump or a power-driven syringe. Many drugs have been given by this route, including meperidine[42] and morphine,[43] and there is little doubt as to the vastly improved analgesia of this method.[44] A steady state can be rapidly achieved with either a bolus dose or a two-rate infusion. Further refinements of the technique have utilized patient-controlled analgesics.[45,46]

Patient-Controlled Analgesia

Patient-controlled analgesia (PCA) pumps allow the patient to self-administer predetermined aliquots of IV narcotic without the assistance of hospital personnel and the attendant delay in analgesia. Theoretically, the patient is (with appropriate drug choice, dosage, and lock-out intervals) able to maintain a plasma level with peaks below the toxic level and troughs above the therapeutic level in a manner similar to that of the ideal IV infusion. Just as inappropriately low or high infusion rates can lead to either subtherapeutic or toxic plasma drug levels, respectively, therapeutic failure can also occur with PCA at either extreme. Subtherapeutic levels result when bolus dosages are set too low or lock-out intervals are too long. Toxic levels often result when less lipophilic drugs are selected in an attempt to increase the duration of action from each aliquot injected. The lag between peak levels in the plasma and CNS may be significant, and if inappropriate short lock-out intervals are selected the patient may inject a second or even third dose before the first dose has achieved maximal effect.

Most PCA devices have the capability of providing a baseline continuous infusion with superimposed additional bolus doses given on patient demand. While this approach has been used with excellent results,[41] recent studies have questioned the added benefit gained with baseline continuous infusions.[47] The need for individually tailored, closely monitored regimes cannot be overemphasized. Wide variation in postsurgical analgesic requirements can be expected owing to preexisting variations in coping styles,[48] psychological factors,[41] and physiological factors such as individual endorphin and substance P levels.[49]

Regional Analgesia

Many of the general constraints discussed previously apply to the use of regionally applied agents such as local anesthetics. In the patient with compromised cardiovascular function, care must be exercised when administering drugs that will have further depressant effects on cardiac or cerebral functions. Routes of administration that produce sympathetic blockade are inappropriate in the hypovolemic patient, which precludes spinal or epidural analgesia until the blood volume is restored to normal. However, the use of regional anesthesia in postthoracotomy patients not only avoids the systemic effects of narcotics but diminishes the stress response. These facts, combined with the completeness of the pain relief afforded by the placement of only a few milliliters of local anesthetic on a nerve, make this technique advantageous.

Local anesthetics can be administered by the following routes: topical (transdermal), infiltration, IV regional, peripheral nerve, and major conduction blockade (epidural or intrathecal; Fig. 4–3). Regional blockade provides excellent analgesia while leaving the patient

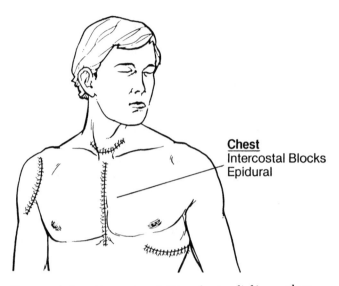

FIGURE 4–3.   Sites and modalities of pain relief in postthoracotomy patients.

awake and cooperative. This might prevent the development of secondary changes that would impair postoperative weaning from mechanical ventilation or lead to a resumption of mechanical ventilatory support after initial postoperative extubation of the trachea.

Intercostal Nerve Blockade

This is indicated for lateral chest wall pain when the pain is in the intercostal nerve distribution. The intercostal nerve block should be one above and one below the site of injury and thus multiple injection sites are required. Intercostal nerve blocks may be particularly difficult at the uppermost thoracic levels where paravertebral blocks may be preferable. Furthermore, intercostal blocks usually are repeated at least twice daily, although analgesia as long as 16 hours has been obtained when bupivacaine is used.[50] There is an increased risk of pneumothorax in such patients. It is possible to insert a catheter into the intercostal space and, by injecting a large volume, block several adjacent segments. This may obviate the need for frequent multiple needle punctures.[51,52]

Interpleural Blockade

Recently, interpleural administration of local anesthetic via a percutaneously placed catheter has been described (Fig. 4–4).[53,54] This technique provides unilateral thoracic analgesia, which is ideally

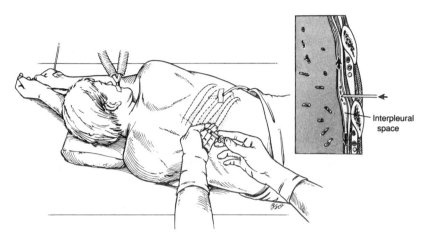

FIGURE 4-4.   Intrapleural block.

suited for patients with unilateral lateral thoracic pain especially with multiple rib fractures.[55] Although the presence of thoracostomy tubes does not preclude use of this technique,[56] it works best in situations where no such drains are required. For median sternotomy, this technique is not suitable as it requires bilateral interpleural block. Even though some clinicians do perform bilateral interpleural blocks, this is not recommended due to increased evidence of systemic toxicity and/or pneumothorax.

When chest tubes are present in unilateral interpleural block, the duration of analgesia following a single instillation usually falls from the expected 10 to 12 hours to less than 4 hours. This effect does not seem to be due to anesthetic egress via the tubes, as it occurs even when the tubes are clamped. Further, with interpleural catheters, one seems to be limited to the bolus mode, as continuous infusion has not been effective. The degree of sensory anesthesia obtained with interpleural block is also inconsistent. Frequently, pinprick sensation is well maintained despite adequate analgesia.

Thoracic Epidural Analgesia

Davis et al. demonstrated in dogs undergoing coronary artery occlusion that thoracic epidural anesthesia decreased the parameters associated with myocardial O_2 consumption, improved regional or ischemic zones of endocardial perfusion, and reduced myocardial infarct size.[57] Blomberg et al. has demonstrated in humans that thoracic epidural anesthesia (TEA) may increase the diameter of stenotic epicardial coronary arteries without dilating coronary arterioles.[58] In patients with severe coronary artery disease and unstable angina, TEA was shown to benefit the determinants of myocardial oxygen consumption without affecting the coronary perfusion pressure.[59] These studies suggest that high-risk patients and patients with known coronary artery disease may exhibit beneficial effects from TEA that greatly exceed the optimal analgesia seen.

Patients undergoing median sternotomy often have multiple system disease and must be classified as high risk. Clearly, it has been shown in clinical studies that high risk patients undergoing nonthoracic surgery benefit from epidural analgesia.[39,60] Why this benefit exists has not been fully elucidated but does extend beyond simply "excellent analgesia."

When analgesia is not adequate in patients suffering rib fractures from trauma, thoracic epidural analgesia with local anesthetic, narcotic, or both may be required. Initially, thoracic epidural was suggested for patients in whom pain was the dominant pathology,[62] but it is now also appreciated that epidural blockade can improve the diminished compliance, increase the vital capacity and functional residual capacity, and decrease the high bronchial resistance seen in these patients.[62,63] This has led to a more aggressive approach to the treatment of rib fractures, based on the recognition that the problem is primarily a functional, rather than an anatomical, derangement.[64,65] Ullman et al. studied patients with multiple rib fractures and reported the use of continuous thoracic epidural narcotic infusion to reduce the subsequent incidence of tracheostomy, reduce the duration of ventilator dependence, and reduce the time spent in both the intensive care unit and hospital.[67] While clinical trials have demonstrated the benefits of postoperative thoracic epidural analgesia, the beneficial effect of regional anesthesia on respiratory complications has been questioned.[67] It remains unclear whether the findings reported for thoracic trauma or lateral thoracotomies will apply to median sternotomies as well. Further investigations of thoracic epidural analgesia after median sternotomy are thus needed.

A thoracic epidural block with local anesthetic should be undertaken with care in a patient who is compromised, and should not be performed until hypovolemia has been corrected. It is recommended that not more than five or six dermatomes be blocked; if more than this number need to be blocked, it should be the lower ribs that are preferentially blocked, as these will interfere less with the cardioaccelerator fibers.[62] Blockade can be maintained with intermittent dosing or continuous infusion; the latter has many of the same advantages previously enumerated with IV narcotic administration and continuous regional blockade.

Effect of Anticoagulation.   There is no absolute answer to the question of the safety of performing epidural anesthesia when coagulation abnormalities exist. Major abnormalities would intuitively preclude the use of regional anesthesia, although controlled studies are lacking.

There have been five studies in which anticoagulation preceded or followed a spinal or epidural anesthetic. No spinal hematomas or neurologic complications were reported. In the first, Matthews and Abrams[68] performed a lumbar puncture on 40 people to deliver intrathecal morphine for open-heart surgery. Fifty minutes later they were heparinized. In the second study, Rao and El-Etr[69] reported on 4,011 people who had either continuous spinal or epidural anesthesia for peripheral vascular surgery. One hour after the anesthetic, heparin was given to increase the activated clotting time to twice baseline. The catheter was left in place for 24 hours postoperatively. In the third study, Odoom and Sih[70] reported on 950 people taking oral anticoagulants, whose preoperative thrombotest was 19% (normal: 70% to 130%). An epidural catheter was placed as the anesthetic technique for vascular surgery, during which the patients were anticoagulated with heparin. In the fourth study, Waldman et al.[71] administered 336 caudal blocks with morphine and bupivacaine to patients with cancer who were either anticoagulated or thrombocytopenic from radiation or chemotherapy. The prothrombin time (PT) or activated partial thromboplastin time (aPTT) was greater than 1.5 times control. The platelet count was less than 50,000. No spinal hematomas or neuralgic complications were reported in any of these four studies. Finally, El Baz reported continuous epidural infusion in 30 patients undergoing cardiac surgery.[72] No epidural hematomas were recorded. All patients had epidural catheters inserted 1 to 2 hours before the administration of heparin for cardiopulmonary bypass.

In clinical practice, a spinal hematoma with neurologic dysfunction is rare from any abnormality of the coagulation system: platelet, anticoagulant, or vascular. Even spontaneous hemorrhage of unknown etiology and traumatic punctures may rarely cause a spinal hematoma. Controversy exists over the exact level of platelet dysfunction or anticoagulation that is safe for the administration of a spinal or epidural anesthetic. However, recent studies suggest that a mild degree of anticoagulation, thrombocytopenia, or platelet dysfunction does not increase the risk of spinal bleeding and hematoma formation, if caution and appropriate timing are used for lumbar puncture or epidural catheter placement and removal, and in monitoring the level of anticoagulation. In a review of the literature, Owen et al. found 33 cases of epidural hematomas after lumbar puncture, and 26 (70%) of these had some type of hemostatic abnormality.[73] These abnormalities included aspirin therapy, thrombocytopenia, heparin and/or coumadin, and idiosyncratic prolonged bleeding time. The denominator from which an accurate incidence can be obtained is impossible to deduce. In combined large series of greater than 50,000 spinal anesthetics, no epidural hematomas were noted.[73]

Intermittent versus Continuous Technique. The *intermittent bolus technique* is often unsatisfactory due to breakthrough pain every few hours, intermittent sympathetic blockade causing hypotension, and the development of tachyphylaxis.[74] Furthermore, the burden of such injections on the medical staff are outside the staffing levels of most hospitals. Continuous infusions offer a much more logical approach from both the pharmacologic and the manpower viewpoints.[75] By adjusting the concentration and the volume of the infusate, one can alter the intensity and extent of the blockade. Once the block has been established, it is often possible to maintain it with a relatively weak solution, minimizing incidence of toxic reaction.

Sternotomy wounds require analgesic spread to include mid-to-upper thoracic dermatomes. For local anesthesia infusion, the catheter tip is best placed near the center of the dermatomal band required. Severe pain can be engendered by regression of the block by as little as one segment, and in the early stages this can occur rapidly. In these cases, addition of a narcotic to the infusate does not detract from the advantages of the local anesthetic agent, but rather improves the analgesia without requiring the use of a dense motor block.

When lipid-soluble narcotics such as fentanyl or meperidine are employed, catheter placement is also quite important, as cephalad migration within the CSF is limited by extensive local uptake.[76–78] However, Melendez et al., in a recent study, have shown that lumbar epidural fentanyl was a safe and practical alternative to thoracic administration.[79] When less lipophilic agents such as morphine are used, catheter placement is less important. The lumbar epidural administration of morphine is often satisfactory for analgesia in even upper thoracic wounds.

Furthermore, the duration of analgesia with bolus administration of lipophilic agents such as fentanyl, sufentanil, or meperidine is less than what is seen with morphine, and these are best administered as an infusion. However, epidural administration of other more lipophilic agents such as buprenorphine may have durations approaching that of morphine because of possible extended receptor binding within the spinal cord.[80,81]

The risk of delayed respiratory depression with intraspinal narcotics seems to increase with thoracic as opposed to lumbar epidural placement, advanced patient age, preexisting pulmonary disease, larger doses, use of water-soluble (less lipophilic) narcotics, and concomitant systemic administration of narcotic.[82,83] Respiratory depression or apnea is usually preceded, however, by increasing sedation.[84] The onset of somnolence should alert the nursing staff to the possibility of impending respiratory depression. Small doses of systemic naloxone or a systemic naloxone infusion (2.5 μg/kg/hr and titrated to effect) reverse respiratory depression without interfering with analgesia.

Adjunctive Measures

Stimulation-induced analgesia, usually using transcutaneous electrical nerve stimulation (TENS),[85] can be effective in reducing acute postsurgical or traumatic pain. Hypnosis has also been used in posttraumatic acute-pain settings with some success.[86] These techniques should be considered as examples of uncommonly used adjunctive measures to supplement the methods previously discussed.

SUMMARY

The pain from median sternotomy can be acute (postoperative) or chronic. Acute pain relief modalities available are similar to those for other postoperative situations. However, clinical studies involving modalities other than intravenous opioids are few, leaving much room for future investigation. Chronic pain syndromes are regionalized to thoracic viscera and somatic structures. Appropriately recognized early, adequate management of such syndromes would decrease the period of suffering and improve their chances of return to normal function.

References

1. Burch GE, Giles TD: Cardiac causalgia. Arch Intern Med 125:809, 1970
2. Simons DG, Travell J: Myofascial trigger points, a possible explanation [letter]. Pain 10:106–109, 1981
3. Bengtsson A, Henriksson KG, Larsson J: Reduced high-energy phosphate levels in the painful muscles of patients with primary fibromyalgia. Arthritis Rheum 29:817–821, 1986

4. Caro XJ: Immunofluorescent detection of IgG at the dermal–epidermal junction in patients with apparent primary fibrositis syndrome. Arthritis Rheum 27:1174–1179, 1984

5. Bonadede P, Nelson D, Clark S, et al: Exercising blood flow in patient with fibrositis: A 113 Xenon clearance study (abstr). Arthritis Rheum 30:S14, 1987

6. Lund N, Bengtsson A, Thorborg P: Muscle tissue oxygen pressure, in primary fibromyalgia. Scand J Rheumatol 15:165–173, 1986

7. Tietze A: Uber eine eigenartige Haufung von Fallen mit Dystrophie der Rippenknorpel. Berl Klin Wochenschr 58:829–831, 1921

8. Fam AG, Smythe HA: Musculoskeletal chest wall pain. Can Med Assoc J 133:379–389, 1985

9. Travell J, Simons DG: Myofascial pain and dysfunction: The trigger point manual, Thoracolombar Paraspinal Muscles pp. 639–659. Baltimore, Williams & Wilkins Co., 1983

10. Bonica JJ: The management of pain. Philadelphia, Lea & Febiger, 1953

11. Wall PD, Devor M: Sensory afferent impulses originate from dorsal root ganglia as well as from the periphery in normal and nerve injured rats. Pain 17:321–339, 1983

12. Cousins MJ, Reeve TS, Glynn CJ et al: Neurolytic lumbar sympathetic blockade: Duration of denervation and relief of rest pain. Anaesth Intensive Care 7:121–135, 1979

13. Bach S, Noreng MF, Tjellden NU: Phantom limb pain in amputees during the first 12 months following limb amputation, after preoperative lumbar epidural blockade. Pain 33:297–301, 1988

14. Melzack R, Abbott FV, Zackon W et al: Pain on a surgical ward: A survey of the duration and intensity of pain and the effectiveness of medication. Pain 29:67–72, 1987

15. Wang JK, Nauss LA, Thomas JE: Pain relief by intrathecally applied morphine in man. Anesthesiology 50:149–151, 1979

16. Cousins MJ: Pathophysiology of acute pain: Immediate and prolonged effects, in Advances in Regional Anesthesia and Analgesia, 2nd International Symposium Regional Anesthesia, pp. 55–56, 1988

17. Tasker RR: Deafferentation. In Wall PD, Melzack R (eds): Textbook of Pain, pp. 119–132. New York, Churchill Livingstone, 1984

18. Hoffert MJ, Greenberg RP, Wolskee PJ et al: Abnormal and collateral innervations of sympathetic and peripheral sensory fields associated with a case of causalgia. Pain 20:1–12, 1984

19. Chahl LA: Pain induced by inflammatory mediators. In Beers RF, Basset EG (eds): Mechanisms of Pain and Analgesic Compounds, pp. 273–284. New York, Raven Press, 1979

20. Cousins MJ: Introduction to acute and chronic pain: Implications for neural blockade. In Cousins MJ, Bridenbaugh PO (eds): Neural Blockade in Clinical Anesthesia and Management of Pain, 2nd ed., pp. 739–752. Philadelphia, J.B. Lippincott Co., 1988

21. Perl ER: Sensitization of nociceptors and its relation to sensation. In Bonica JJ, Albe-Fessard D (eds): Advances in Pain Research and Therapy, vol 1, pp. 17–28. New York, Raven Press, 1976

22. Kelley JT: Chronic pain and trauma. Adv Psychosom Med 16:141–142, 1986

23. Benedikt RA, Kolb LC: Preliminary findings on chronic pain and post-traumatic stress disorder. Am J Psychiatry 143:908–910, 1986
24. Fields HL: Sources of variability in the sensation of pain. Pain 33:195–200, 1988
25. Rosenfeld JP, Silvia R, Weitkunat R et al: Operant control of human somatosensory evoked potentials alters experimental pain perception. In Fields HL et al (eds): Advances in Pain Research and Therapy, vol 9, pp. 343–349. New York, Raven Press, 1985
26. Duncan GH, Bushnell MC, Bates R et al: Task-related responses of monkey medullary dorsal horn neurons. J Neurophysiol 59:289–310, 1987
27. Cooper JD, Nelems JM, Pearson FG: Extended indications for median sternotomy in patients requiring pulmonary resection. Ann Thorac Surg 26:413–420, 1978
28. Mattila T, Laustela E, Talla P: On the effect of sternotomy and thoracotomy incision on pulmonary function after open-heart operations. Ann Chir Gynaecol Fenn 56:58–61, 1967
29. Peters RM, Wellons HA, Htwe TM: Total compliance and work of breathing after thoracotomy. J Thorac Cardiovasc Surg 57:348–355, 1969
30. Howatt WF, Talner NS, Sloan H, DeMuth GR: Pulmonary function changes following repair of heart lesions with the aid of extracorporeal circulation. J Thorac Cardiovasc Surg 43:649–657, 1962
31. Tarhan S, Moffitt EA, Sessler AD, Douglas WW, Taylor WF: Risk of anesthesia and surgery in patients with chronic bronchitis and chronic obstructive pulmonary disease. Surgery 74:720–726, 1973
32. Ali J, Weisel RD, Layug AB, Kripke BJ, Hechtman HB: Consequences of postoperative alterations in respiratory mechanics. Am J Surg 128:376–382, 1974
33. Cousins MJ, Wright CJ: Graft, muscle, skin blood flow after epidural block in vascular surgical procedures. Surg Gynecol Obstet 133:59–69, 1971
34. Bridenbaugh PO: Anesthesia and influence on hospitalization time. Reg Anaesth [Suppl] 7:S151–155, 1982
35. Noller DW, Gillenwater JY et al: Intercostal nerve block with flank incision. J Urol 117:759, 1977
36. Pflug AE, Murphy TM, Butler SH et al: The effects of postoperative peridural analgesic on pulmonary therapy and pulmonary complications. Anesthesiology 41:8–17, 1974
37. Nimmo WS, Littlewood DG, Scott DB et al: Gastric emptying following hysterectomy with extradural analgesia. Br J Anaesth 50:559–561, 1978
38. Shulman M, Sandler AN, Bradley JW et al: Postthoracotomy pain and pulmonary function following epidural and systemic morphine. Anesthesiology 61:569–575, 1984
39. Yeager MP, Glass DD, Neff RK, Brick-Johnsen T: Epidural anesthesia and analgesia in high-risk surgical patients. Anesthesiology 66:729–736, 1987
40. Churchill-Davidson HC: A Practice of Anaesthesia, 4th ed. Philadelphia, W.B. Saunders Co., 1978
41. Gourlay GK, Kowalski SR, Plummer JL et al: Fentanyl blood concentration—Analgesic response relationship in the treatment of postoperative pain. Anesth Analg 67:329–337, 1988

42. Stapleton JV, Austin KL, Mather LE: A pharmacokinetic approach to postoperative pain: Conscious infusion of peridine. Anaesth Intensive Care 7:25–36, 1979

43. Orr IA, Keenan DJ, Dundee JW: Improved pain relief after thoracotomy: Use of cryoprobe and morphine infusion. Br Med J 283:945–948, 1981

44. Mather LE: Parenteral opiates for postoperative analgesia. Reg Anaesth 7:144, 1982

45. Evans JM, MacCarthy J, Rosen M et al: Apparatus for patient controlled administration of intravenous narcotics during labor. Lancet 1:17, 1976

46. Hull CJ, Sibbald A: Control of postoperative pain by interactive demand analgesia. Br J Anaesth 53:385–391, 1981

47. Parker RK, Holtmann B, White PF: Patient-controlled analgesia: Does a concurrent opioid infusion improve pain management after surgery? JAMA 266:1947–1952, 1991

48. Wilson JF, Bennett RL: Coping styles, medication use, and pain score in patients using patient controlled analgesia for postoperative pain. Anesthesiology 61:A193, 1984

49. Tamsen A, Sakurada T, Wahlstrom A et al: Postoperative demand for analgesics in relation to individual levels of endorphins and substance P in cerebrospinal fluid. Pain 13:171–183, 1982

50. Telivou L, Perttala Y: Use of x-ray contrast medium to control intercostal nerve blocks. Ann Chir Gynaecol Fenn 55:185, 1966

51. O'Kelly E, Garry B: Continuous pain relief for multiple fractured ribs. Br J Anaesth 53:987–991, 1981

52. Murphy DF: Intercostal nerve blockade for fractured ribs and postoperative analgesia. Reg Anaesth 8:151–153, 1983

53. Reiestad F, Stromskag KE: Interpleural catheter in the management of postoperative pain. Reg Anaesth 11:89–91, 1986

54. Seltzer JL, Larijani GE, Goldberg ME et al: Intrapleural bupivacaine— A kinetic and dynamic evaluation. Anesthesiology 67:798–800, 1987

55. Rocco A, Reiestad F, Gudman J et al: Intrapleural administration of local anesthetics for pain relief in patients with multiple rib fractures. Reg Anaesth 12:10–14, 1987

56. Lee VC, Abram SE: Interpleural administration of bupivacaine for postthoracotomy analgesia. Anesthesiology 66:586, 1987

57. Davis RF, DeBoer LWV, Maroko PR: Thoracic epidural anesthesia reduces myocardial infarct size after coronary artery occlusion in dogs. Anesth Analg 65:711–717, 1986

58. Blomberg S, Emanuelsson H, Dvist H, Lamm C, Pontén J, Waagstein F, Ricksten S–E: Effects of thoracic epidural anesthesia on coronary arteries and arterioles in patients with coronary artery disease. Anesthesiology 73:840–847, 1990

59. Blomberg S, Emanuelsson H, Ricksten S–E: Thoracic epidural anesthesia and central hemodynamics in patients with unstable angina pectoris. Anesth Analg 69:558–562, 1989

60. Rawal N, Sjostrand U, Christoffersson E, Dahlstrom B, Arvill A, Rydman H: Comparison of intramuscular and epidural morphine for post-

operative analgesia in the grossly obese: Influence on postoperative ambulation and pulmonary function. Anesth Analg 63:583–592, 1984

61. Gibbons J, James O, Quail A: The relief of pain in chest injury. Br J Anaesth 45:1136, 1975

62. Lloyd JW, Rucklidge MA: The management of closed chest injuries. Br J Surg 56:721, 1967

63. Dittman M, Keller R, Wolff G: A rationale for epidural analgesia in the treatment of multiple rib fractures. Intensive Care Med 4:193, 1976

64. Johnson JR, McCaughey GJ: Epidural morphine: A method of management of multiple fractured ribs. Anaesthesia 35:155, 1980

65. Dittman M, Steenblock G, Kranzlin M et al: Epidural analgesia or mechanical ventilation for multiple fractures. Intensive Care Med 8:89–92, 1982

66. Ullman DA, Fortune JB, Greenhouse BB et al: The treatment of patients with multiple rib fractures using continuous thoracic epidural narcotic infusion. Reg Anaesth 14:43–47, 1989

67. Jayr C et al: Postoperative pulmonary complications: General anaesthesia with postoperative parenteral morphine compared with epidural analgesia. Surgery 104:63, 1988

68. Matthews ET, Abrams LD: Intrathecal morphine in open heart surgery. Lancet ii:543, 1980

69. Rao TLK, El-Etr AA: Anticoagulation following placement of epidural and subarachnoid catheters: An evaluation of neurologic sequelae. Anesthesiology 55:618–620, 1981

70. Odoom JA, Sih IL: Epidural analgesia and anticoagulant therapy: Experience with one thousand cases of continuous epidurals. Anaesthesia 38:254–259, 1983

71. Waldman SD, Feldstein GS, Waldman HJ et al: Caudal administration of morphine sulfate in anticoagulated and thrombocytopenic patients. Anesth Analg 66:267–268, 1987

72. El-Baz N, Goldin M: Continuous epidural infusion of morphine for pain relief after cardiac operations. J Thorac Cardiovasc Surg 93:878–883, 1987

73. Owens EL, Kasten GW, Hessel EA: Spinal subarachnoid hematoma after lumbar puncture and heparinization: A case report, review of the literature, and discussion of anesthetic implications. Anesth Analg 65:1201–1207, 1986

74. Bromage PR, Pettigrew RT, Crowell DE: Tachyphylaxis in epidural analgesia. Augmentation and decay of local analgesia. J Clin Pharmacol 9:30, 1969

75. Raj PP, Finnsson R, Denson D: Epidural analgesia—Intermittent or continuous? In Meyer J, Nolte H (eds): Die kontiniuerliche Periduralanasthesie, pp. 26–37. Stuttgart, Georg Thieme Verlag, 1983

76. Moore RA, Bullingham RES, McQuay HJ et al: Dural permeability to narcotics: In vitro determination and application to extradural administration. Br J Anaesth 54:1117–1128, 1982

77. Gourlay GK, Cherry DA, Plummer JL et al: The influence of drug polarity on the absorption of opioid drugs into CSF and subsequent cephalad migration following lumbar epidural administration: Application to morphine and pethidine. Pain 31:297–306, 1987

78. Ahuja BR, Strunin L: Respiratory effects of epidural fentanyl. Anaesthesia 40:949–955, 1985
79. Melendez JA, Cirella VN, Delphin ES: Lumbar epidural fentanyl analgesia after thoracic surgery. J Cardiothorac Anesth 3(2):150–153, 1989
80. Hambrook JM, Rance MJ: The interaction of buprenorphine with opiate receptor: Lipophilicity as a determining factor in drug-receptor kinetics. In Kosterlitz HW (ed): Opiates and Endogenous Opiate Peptides, pp. 295–301. Amsterdam, North-Holland, 1976
81. Kotob HIM, Hand CW, Moore RA et al: Intrathecal morphine and heroin in humans: Six-hour drug levels in spinal fluid and plasma. Anesth Analg 65:718–722, 1986
82. Cousins MJ, Mather LE: Intrathecal and epidural administration of opiates. Anesthesiology 61:276–310, 1984
83. Bromage PR: Clinical aspects of intrathecal and epidural opiates. In Fields HL (ed): Advances in Pain Research and Therapy, vol 9, pp. 733–748. New York, Raven Press, 1985
84. Ready LB, Oden R, Chadwick HS et al: Development of an anesthesiology-based postoperative pain management service. Anesthesiology 68:100–106, 1988
85. Ordog GJ: Transcutaneous electrical nerve stimulation versus oral analgesic: A randomized double-blind controlled study in acute traumatic pain. Am J Emerg Med 5:6–10, 1987
86. Wain HJ, Amen DG: Emergency room use of hypnosis. Gen Hosp Psychiatry 8:19–22, 1986
87. Lynn AM, Slattery JT: Morphine pharmacokinetics in early infancy. Anesthesiology 66:136–139, 1987
88. Bhat R, Chari G, Gulati A et al: Pharmacokinetics of a single dose of morphine in preterm infants during the first week of life. J Pediatr 117:477–481, 1990
89. Dahlstrom B, Bolme P, Feychting H et al: Morphine kinetics in children. Clin Pharmacol Ther 26(3):354–365, 1979
90. Glare PA, Walsh TD: Clinical pharmacokinetics of morphine. Ther Drug Monit 13(1):1–23, 1991
91. Hoskin PJ, Hanks GW, Aherne GW, Chapman D, Littleton P, Filshie J: The bioavailability and pharmacokinetics of morphine after intravenous, oral and buccal administration in healthy volunteers. Br J Clin Pharmacol 27(4):499–505, 1989
92. Dahlstrom B, Tamsen A, Paalzow L, Hartvig P: Patient-controlled analgesic therapy, Part IV: Pharmacokinetics and analgesic plasma concentrations of morphine. Clin Pharmacokinet 7(3):266–279, 1982
93. Garrett ER, Chandran VR: Pharmacokinetics of morphine and its surrogates VI: Bioanalysis, solvolysis kinetics, solubility, pKa values, and protein binding of buprenorphine. J Pharm Sci 74(5):515–524, 1985
94. Inturrisi CE, Colburn WA, Kaiko RF, Houde RW, Foley KM: Pharmacokinetics and pharmacodynamics of methadone in patients with chronic pain. Clin Pharmacol Ther 41(4):392–401, 1987
95. Meresaar U, Nilsson MI, Holmstrand J, Anggard E: Single dose pharmacokinetics and bioavailability of methadone in man studied with a stable isotope method. Eur J Clin Pharmacol 20(6):473–478, 1981

96. Schleimer R, Benjamini E, Eisele J, Henderson G: Pharmacokinetics of fentanyl as determined by radioimmunoassay. Clin Pharmacol Ther 23(2):188–194, 1978

97. Greeley WJ, de Bruijn NP, Davis DP: Sufentanil pharmacokinetics in pediatric cardiovascular patients. Anesth Analg 66(11):1067–1072, 1987

98. Chauvin M, Lebrault C, Levron JC, Duvaldestin P: Pharmacokinetics of alfentanil in chronic renal failure. Anesth Analg 66(1):53–56, 1987

99. Koren G, Goresky G, Crean P, Klein J, MacLeod SM: Pediatric fentanyl dosing based on pharmacokinetics during cardiac surgery. Anesth Analg 63(6):577–582, 1984

100. Shafer A, Sung ML, White PF: Pharmacokinetics and pharmacodynamics of alfentanil infusions during general anesthesia. Anesth Analg 65(10):1021–1028, 1986

101. Koehntop DE, Rodman JH, Brundage DM, Hegland MG, Buckley JJ: Pharmacokinetics of fentanyl in neonates. Anesth Analg 65(3):227–232, 1986

102. Camu F, Gepts E, Rucquoi M, Heykants J: Pharmacokinetics of alfentanil in man. Anesth Analg 61(8):657–661, 1982

103. Bentley JB, Borel JD, Nenad RE Jr, Gillespie TJ: Age and fentanyl pharmacokinetics. Anesth Analg 61(12):968–971, 1982

104. Chauvin M, Ferrier C, Haberer JP, Spielvogel C, Lebrault C, Levron JC, Duvaldestin P: Sufentanil pharmacokinetics in patients with cirrhosis. Anesth Analg 68(1):1–4, 1989

105. Bovill JG, Sebel PS, Blackburn CL, Oei-Lim V, Heykants JJ: The pharmacokinetics of sufentanil in surgical patients. Anesthesiology 61(5):502–506, 1984

106. Goresky GV, Koren G, Sabourin MA, Sale JP, Strunin L: The pharmacokinetics of alfentanil in children. Anesthesiology 67(5):654–659, 1987

107. Bovill JG, Sebel PS, Blackburn CL, Heykants J: The pharmacokinetics of alfentanil (R39209): A new opioid analgesic. Anesthesiology 57(6):439–443, 1982

108. Meisterlman C, Saint-Maurice C, Lepaul M, Levron JC, Loose JP, Mac Gee K: A comparison of alfentanil pharmacokinetics in children and adults. Anesthesiology 66(1):13–16, 1987

109. Hudson RJ, Bergstrom RG, Thomson IR, Sabourin MA, Rosenbloom M, Strunin L: Pharmacokinetics of sufentanil in patients undergoing abdominal aortic surgery. Anesthesiology 70(3):426–431, 1989

110. Hudson RJ, Thomson IR, Cannon JE, Friesen RM, Meatherall RC: Pharmacokinetics of fentanyl in patients undergoing abdominal aortic surgery. Anesthesiology 64(3):334–338, 1986

111. Guay J, Gaudreault P, Tang A, Goulet B, Varin F: Pharmacokinetics of sufentanil in normal children. Can J Anaesth 39(1):14–20, 1992

112. Roure P, Jean N, Leclerc AC, Cabanel N, Levron JC, Duvaldestin P: Pharmacokinetics of alfentanil in children undergoing surgery. Br J Anaesth 59(11):1437–1440, 1987

113. Matteo RS, Schwartz AE, Ornstein E, Young WL, Chang W: Pharmacokinetics of sufentanil in the elderly surgical patient. Can J Anaesth 37(8):852–856, 1990

114. Duthie DJ, McLaren AD, Nimmo WS: Pharmacokinetics of fentanyl

during constant rate i.v. infusion for the relief of pain after surgery. Br J Anaesth 58(9):950–956, 1986

115. Chauvin M, Salbaing J, Perrin D, Levron JC, Viars P: Clinical assessment and plasma pharmacokinetics associated with intramuscular or extradural alfentanil. Br J Anaesth 57(9):886–891, 1985

116. Van Beem H, Van Peer A, Gasparini R, Woestenborghs R, Heykants J, Noorduin H, Van Egmond J, Crul J: Pharmacokinetics of alfentanil during and after a fixed rate infusion. Br J Anaesth 62(6):610–615, 1989

117. Singleton MA, Rosen JI, Fisher DM: Pharmacokinetics of fentanyl in the elderly. Br J Anaesth 60(6):619–622, 1988

118. Scott JC, Stanski DR: Decreased fentanyl and alfentanil dose requirements with age. A simultaneous pharmacokinetic and pharmacodynamic evaluation J Pharmacol Exp Ther 240(1):159–166, 1987

119. Shafer SL, Varvel JR: Pharmacokinetics, pharmacodynamics and rational opioid selection. Anesthesiology 74:53–63, 1991

120. David PT, Cook DR, Stiller RL, Davin-Robinson KA: Pharmacodynamics and pharmacokinetics of high-dose sufentanil in infants and children undergoing cardiac surgery. Anesthesiology 66:203–208, 1987

121. Gauntlett IS, Fisher DM, Hertzka RE, Kuhis E, Spellman MJ, Rudolph C: Pharmacokinetics of fentanyl in neonatal humans and lambs: Effects of age. Anesthesiology 69:683–687, 1988

122. Gourlay GK, Wilson PR, Glynn CJ: Pharmacodynamics and pharmacokinetics of methadone during the perioperative period. Anesthesiology 57:458–467, 1982

123. Greeley WJ, de Bruijn NP: Changes in sufentanil pharmacokinetics within the neonatal period. Anesth Analg 67:86–90, 1988

124. Baillie SP, Bateman DN, Coates PE, Woodhouse KW: Age and the pharmacokinetics of morphine. Age and Aging 18:258–262, 1989

125. Mather LE: Clinical pharmacokinetics of fentanyl and its newer derivatives. Clin Pharmacokinet 8:422–446, 1983

126. Bower S, Hull CJ: Comparative pharmacokinetics of fentanyl and alfentanil. Br J Anaesth 54:871–877, 1982

127. Halliburton JR: The pharmacokinetics of fentanyl, sufentanil and alfentanil: A comparative review. J Am Assoc Nur Anesth 56(3):229–233, 1988

Pain Management in Cardiothoracic Surgery, edited by Gravlee and Rauck. J. B. Lippincott Company, Philadelphia © 1993.

David A. Rosen
Kathleen R. Rosen

5 | Pain Control for Pediatric Cardiac and Thoracic Surgery

No one, children included, enjoys being a consumer in a hospital, where the environment is characterized by numerous anxiety-provoking events and people. Children often respond negatively to even small variations in their routine. In the hospital, the child is removed from the comfort and security of home and may even be separated from friends and family. White coats and uniforms, disinfectant odors, and a strange and uncomfortable bed are the unwelcome replacements. Older children who appreciate causal relationships fear coming into the hospital because of the inevitable pain and discomfort required for diagnosis and treatment. Hospitals can impact significantly on a child's behavior. Children who have recently reached developmental milestones frequently regress following hospitalization. Pain experienced as a result of medical intervention can produce serious, long-term psychological effects.[1] Fear of pain and distrust of health providers may be evident into adulthood, potentially interfering with the acquisition of preventive or even urgent health care.

The focus of modern medicine tends to be problem-oriented rather than process-oriented. The primary presenting complaint for many patients is pain. Despite the prevalence and longevity of pain, methods for the detection and treatment of this problem are often archaic compared to those used for many less common and less obvious symptoms.

125

A pain awareness and management renaissance occurred during the 1980s, and pain became a frequent topic in the popular press. As the general public becomes more educated about pain and pain relief options, patients less often are willing to tolerate traditional approaches. There are still many missing links in the basic medical knowledge about pain. Pain theories abound but none effectively answers all the questions. Although the forward strides undertaken with adult pain management are impressive, many of the old concepts and pain myths unfortunately persist in pediatric practice. The experience of pain in infants and children is often devalued and the risks of effective pain control are exaggerated. One problem is that verbal skills are essential to many pain assessment and management scales, thus it is impossible to utilize these scales with small children.

A review of the medical literature reveals limited information on pediatric pain management. Early studies typically reported only the incidence of pain medication administration. In 1968, Swafford and Allan documented that only 26 of 180 children received postoperative narcotics in an intensive care setting.[2] Beyer[3,4] was the first to compare postoperative pain relief in children and adults undergoing similar major surgical procedures. Following cardiac surgery with cardiopulmonary bypass, analgesics were prescribed for all adults sampled, but for only 44 of 50 children. During the first three postoperative days adult patients received a mean of 10 doses while children received only 3.2 doses, and a non-narcotic option was frequently selected in children but not adults. Furthermore, 50% of the analgesic prescriptions for children fell below the therapeutic range when indexed for age and weight. In 1983, Mather and Mackie became the first authors who asked children about the quality of pain control resulting from the prescribed regimen.[5] They found that the majority of children noted moderate or severe pain despite the analgesic prescription. By 1989, the situation had improved slightly, but differences persisted, with Schecter reporting that adults received 1.5 to 3 times as many analgesic doses per day as children undergoing similar surgical procedures.[6]

Currently, there are several islands of hope for standards of care for the child in pain. A prototype multidisciplinary approach to pain management in children at Boston Children's Hospital has spurred the development of similar resources nationwide. Epidural opiates and patient-controlled analgesia have become clinical options rather than research techniques.

However, optimism is dampened by a 1992 survey from Yale University that describes the persistent inadequacy of pain relief in children undergoing cardiac surgery.[7] Intravenous morphine at a dose of 0.1 mg/kg was ordered every 3 hours. Although the route, frequency, and dosage were shown to be much improved compared to prescriptions of only a decade earlier, a lack of understanding about pediatric narcotic pharmacology was evident. Pharmacokinetics vary with age and disease state. Further, this report indicated that even in the controlled environment of an ICU, the nurses still feared the use of opiates in children to such a degree that needed medication was withheld.

PAIN CONTROL DIFFICULTIES

Pediatric Pain Myths

For many years the rationale for inadequate treatment of pain in children was the mistaken belief that children cannot experience pain due to immaturity of the central and peripheral nervous systems. Anand and colleagues recently reviewed the convincing anatomic and physiologic evidence that even premature neonates can feel pain.[8,9] The cutaneous sensory receptors develop between the 7th and 20th week of gestation. The density of these fibers may be even greater in the neonate than in the adult. The next important phase in pain perception is the development of neocortex, which occurs from weeks 8 to 20. The cortical synapses then develop (weeks 20–24) followed by the initiation of clinical brain function (week 28). The nervous system is then completely functional, but it becomes more efficient with myelination. Myelination begins in the brain stem and thalamus followed by the thalamocortical tracts. Only the peripheral nervous system myelinates after birth. The very short distance that a pain impulse must travel in an infant counteracts the effect of incomplete myelination. At birth, neonates do show elevated plasma levels of beta endorphins, but these levels fall far short of concentrations that would be required to produce analgesia, and they return to baseline by 24 days of age.[10,11] Pain system development continues in older children and adolescents, and psychologic effects of pain develop, including the meaning of pain, affective components of pain, integration with memory of previous events, and pain associated behaviors.

Chameleon Nature of Pain

It is apparent from the work done by Anand that even the preterm infant is capable of experiencing pain. However, pain is not always easily identified or outwardly apparent. Children may express pain, anxiety, fear, and anger all in a similar fashion. Pain is a very individual experience, and its intensity and perception is different for every child. Pain will often be overlooked if it is not specifically investigated, because it is not always possible to differentiate pain from other sources of psychic and physiologic distress. Sometimes we do not find out that there was pain until after it is treated.

Comparison Inadequacies

Zeltzer has classified children into four groups according to their response to pain and their ability to cope with it.[12] The first group is labeled pain vulnerable. These children have a low threshold for pain and poorly developed coping mechanisms. The second, the highly reactive group, also has a low threshold for pain, but the child's adaptive capabilities enhance effective pain measures. The third, low reactive group has a higher threshold for pain but when this threshold is exceeded, they are poorly adaptive. The final group is pain resilient. A high threshold for pain and the presence of facilitative adaptive behavior enhances pharmacologic and other methods of pain control. It does not appear that we can change a child from one group to another, nor should we try, thus a cookbook approach will not work for all children. Identification of the group can help us prepare for what lies ahead. The cold pressor pain paradigm measures the child's response to placing an arm in cold water. This model allows testing of interventional strategies and allows characterization of the child's response to pain.[13] If a system like this were utilized prior to the onset of pain, it could facilitate development of a pain management strategy.

Limitations of Pain Research

Because pain is a subjective, multidimensional experience, it is difficult to quantify and compare. Many pain assessment techniques rely heavily on the patient's ability to describe and verbalize pain and, therefore, are not useful with infants and children. A number of tools have been developed which incorporate the physiologic, behavioral, and psychologic aspects of pain. Although these are imperfect, they should be utilized until better alternatives are developed.[14]

The majority of studies on children in pain rely on the presence, absence, or frequency of analgesics administered as the sole measure of pain treatment. The examination of pain treatment, in terms of drug delivery alone, is incomplete. The quality of pain control achieved with the prescribed regimen is also very important. Most of the studies, especially those that focus on cardiacthoracic postoperative pain relief reviewed in this chapter, describe the experience with adult patients. These studies are frequently descriptive in nature and present a "how I do it" approach to pain relief. We have attempted to extract the key points of these studies and apply them to the pediatric patient. Comparative studies, which compare specific pain relief techniques, are very limited involving children.

Exaggerated Fear of Opiate Addiction in Children

Parents are informed of the hazards of drug dependence and children are admonished to "just say no." Problems associated with the illicit use of opioids and other controlled substances are irrelevant when their monitored use is indicated in a medical environment. However irrational it may be when opiates are used for short-term control of acute pain, fear of addiction persists among both families and medical personnel.[3] Further, many drug awareness programs now in place in school systems fail to adequately differentiate the use of these medications. Many of the studies of current analgesic practice report these fears as the primary rationalization for inadequate medication of patients in pain. Respiratory depression can be minimized by knowledge of the pharmacology and appropriate patient monitoring. Table 5–1 summarizes some of the currently available pharmacokinetic data for analgesics as a function of age. By appreciating the changes in pharmacokinetics as the child ages, rational dosing plans can be developed.

Time Consuming Nature of Pain Control

Restricted access to controlled substances increases the workload of health care professionals. On a postoperative care ward, each nurse will spend more than 8 hours of a 40-hour work week obtaining and

TABLE 5-1. Pharmacokinetic Data Obtained from a Large Number of Sources Listed in Reference Section as Letters. See References 15–55

Drug	Age	Distribution Half Life (Minutes)	Elimination Half Life (Hours)	Clearance (ml/kg/min)	V_D (L/KG)	V_DSS	Protein Binding (%)	MEC NG/ML
Alfentanil	Preterm		8.75	2.2	1	0.55		
	Term		1	5.5	0.48	0.42		
	Children	3.5	.75	7.9	0.42	0.996	89	
	Adults		1.2	7.5	0.28	0.277	89	300
	Aged Adults		1.95	1.8			85–89	<Adults
Fentanyl	Preterm		17.1					
	Neonates		4.9	18.4	5.1			
	Infants	12	4	11.5	3.06			
	Children	12	3.5	7.05	1.92			
	Adults	5–12	1–4	12.8	4.7	2.2	43–80	20
	Aged Adults		15.75	3.5		1.4		
Meperidine	Infants			10.4	3.74			
	Adults		2.3	2.7	1.1			
Methadone	Adults	6.1	35	3.39		6.1		
	<30 weeks	50	10					
Morphine	Term	19	6.7	15	3.38			
	Infants		3.9	5.2	23.8		18	
	Children			23.8	10.4		22	12
	Adult		2	11.5	6	1–3	30	16
	Adult Post Op		2.2		3.7		35	
	Aged Adults			13.3	5.5			
Sufentanil	Neonate	20.5	12.7	6.7	4.15	2.7		2.5
	Infants	15.8	3.6	18.1	2.73	3.4		4.58
	Children	5.2–19.6	2.3	16.9	2.75	2.9		1.5
	Adolescents	20.4	3.5	13.1	2.75	2.8		1.56
	Adults	17	3.5	11.3	2.9	1.7	61–91	
	Aged Adults			15	<Adult	8.7		

delivering narcotics. Several steps are involved, including paperwork and a witness signature. In the pediatric patient, this may be exacerbated if adult preparations are used, because the additional step of obtaining a witness to the waste of excess narcotic is needed. These time-consuming processes may encourage nurses to select a noncontrolled analgesic option when one is available. Similarly, for busy physicians, follow-up is a time-consuming, low-priority, and often unrewarding activity.

BENEFITS OF PAIN CONTROL

Compassion should be incentive enough to strive for adequate pain control in pediatric patients, but a large number of caregivers allow their fears to predominate. Untreated pathologic pain, like that produced by surgery, results in a cascade of detrimental physiologic and psychological effects. The stress response triggered by pain is characterized by vasoconstriction, elevated catecholamines, hypercoagulability, immunosuppression, and a general catabolic state.[56] These changes can manifest clinically as increased weight loss, poor feeding, delayed healing, postoperative infections, tachycardia, hypertension, or irritability.

Several reports document positive outcomes associated with improved pain control.[57] Semsroth and Hiesmayr studied oxygen consumption in response to two different types of pain management in intubated children after cardiac surgery.[58] This study compared intravenous morphine by intermittent bolus to continuous infusion. The group receiving a continuous infusion of morphine at 0.1–1 mcg/kg/min had lower oxygen consumption than the intermittent bolus group (0.05 mg/kg) given as needed. Although the groups had no difference in pain scores, oxygen consumption was decreased in groups receiving continuous pain relief. They concluded that continuous infusion represented stress prevention while intermittent bolus represented stress treatment.

Pain limits respiratory volumes, which are essential to postoperative recovery and the prevention of pulmonary infection.[59] The substitution of quality pain relief significantly lowered the $PaCO_2$ in children with thoracic pain. Ninety percent of adult patients undergoing cardiac surgery develop left lower lobe atelectasis during the immediate postoperative period.[60] Following surgical repair of congenital heart disease in children the incidence of atelectasis is also high, but the severity of the atelectasis has been improved with attention to quality pain control.[61] Diaphragmatic dysfunction represents one proposed mechanism for the postoperative respiratory changes seen in patients undergoing thoracic and cardiac surgery. This may be caused by trauma to the diaphragm, phrenic nerves, or autonomic system. The involvement of the autonomic system may be through the respiratory center, which receives an increase in phrenic nerve-inhibitory afferent activity conducted by medullary pathways. This decreases diaphragmatic activity as evidenced by a decrease in the electrical activity of costal and crural fibers. The exact mechanism remains unclear but epidural analgesia can reduce the diaphragmatic dysfunction.[62]

Poor outcomes, including death, may be attributed to inadequate pain control, but it is difficult to prove that pain is the sole or major determinant. Parfey found a higher incidence of unexplained death during sickle cell crises, in children who were in pain when compared to those who were pain free.[63] Several studies imply that anesthesia and pain management can profoundly affect morbidity and mortality in the neonate.[64–69] In children undergoing major surgery, the lowest mortality was observed in the patients who received the most complete analgesia. Anand contrasted neonates who received a halothane anesthetic followed by morphine on a p.r.n. basis to neonates who received a high-dose sufentanil anesthetic technique, followed by a postoperative sufentanil or fentanyl infusion postoperatively. Mortality was significantly lower in the group receiving the narcotic infusion. In addition, the halothane–morphine group experienced more hyperglycemia, higher levels of lactate and acetate, as well as more frequent sepsis, disseminated intravascular coagulation, and metabolic acidosis. The maintenance of intraoperative narcotic levels appears to be beneficial. A recent study indicates that neonates undergoing open cardiac surgery for correction of hypoplastic left heart syndrome had lower mortality when fentanyl plasma levels were maintained above 20 ng/ml throughout the surgical procedure.[28] In this study, the control group patients received only a bolus of fentanyl (50–100 mcg/kg) at the beginning of the case. The experimental group received a smaller bolus (35 mcg/kg) followed by a continuous infusion of fentanyl (0.3 mcg/kg/min). Further, the experimental group had the cardiopulmonary bypass circuit loaded with sufficient fentanyl to saturate the SciMed membrane oxygenator (130 ng/square cm membrane), while the control group did not. Because of the oxygenator membrane (SciMed) uptake, fentanyl levels decreased during cardiopulmonary bypass in the control group, while they remained above 20 ng/ml in the experimental group.[69] This degree of fentanyl uptake appears unique to the silicone-type (SciMed) membrane oxygenate.

POSTOPERATIVE PAIN

Postoperative pain is often de-emphasized in relationship to the structural, functional, and hemodynamic changes that characterize the surgical procedure. The surgical approach influences postoperative pain, as noted by an increase in postoperative pain and analgesic requirements when the same corrective procedure is performed through a lateral thoracotomy as compared to a sternotomy.[70] Asaph and Keppel found that thoracotomy patients required narcotic analgesics long after patients with sternotomies had converted to nonnarcotic analgesics. On the sixth postoperative day almost 50% of patients who had thoracotomy incisions still requested narcotic analgesics.[70] Although these data were derived from adult patients, our experience with children are similar. Correction of an atrial septal defect through a thoracotomy is associated with increased morphine dosage requirements for an extended duration.

NONSURGICAL CARDIAC PAIN IN CHILDREN

Cardiac pain may be produced by a variety of mechanisms including structural abnormalities, myopericardial disease, dysrhythmias, or coronary artery disease.[71] Most retrospective studies on children with congenital heart disease do not consider alternative structural sources of chest pain such as ischemia.[71] Pain resulting from acquired myopericardial disease (primary pericardial irritation, myocarditis, cardiomyopathy, etc.) is better recognized and accepted. These processes need to be differentiated from surgical pain because of their extended duration and potentially chronic pain characteristics. Dysrhythmias may produce ischemia, or a more subjective discomfort related to the irregularity of palpitations or aberrant heartbeats. Potential contributors to myocardial ischemia in the postoperative period include stress from incisional and other surgical pain, anxiety related to the ICU setting, separation from family, and feeding. It is important to remember that feeding is a very strenuous activity for an infant that is equivalent to exercise in an adult.

Isolated coronary ischemia is relatively rare in children except when associated with rare familial lipid disorders or coronary venous sinusoids. Coronary venous sinusoids develop in response to right ventricular outflow obstruction and elevated right ventricular pressures. The sinusoidal interconnections promote retrograde coronary artery filling during systole that may well result in ischemia. Children with pulmonic stenosis and an intact ventricular septum can develop ischemic pain by this mechanism.

Congenital anomalies of the coronary arteries are uncommon but can cause cardiac pain in children. Anomalous origin of the coronary arteries often presents in infancy by the sudden unexplained onset of myocardial insufficiency. Pain as a symptom of an anomalous coronary artery would be expected to occur preoperatively. These infants are frequently "colicky babies" and much of their pain is associated with feeding. Occasionally, anomalous coronary arteries are not discovered until the time of repair or recovery from an unrelated congenital cardiac lesion. For example, consider the physiology of a child with a concurrent ductus arteriosus and an anomalous left coronary artery. Preoperatively, oxygenated blood is available to the coronary artery by means of left to right shunt flow through the ductus arteriosus. When the ductus is ligated, the coronary artery will be perfused solely with the desaturated venous return. Ischemic pain may develop postoperatively but be discounted as normal postoperative pain. Aberration of coronary blood flow is also seen when the left coronary artery arises anomalously from the anterior sinus of Valsalva and courses between the aorta and pulmonary artery. During periods of high-cardiac output or elevated intravascular volume, the great vessels are distended and can impede coronary blood flow.[72] Location and radiation of chest pain may be the only indication that the pain is ischemic in origin. Radiation of pain to the neck, jaw, upper extremities, back, or abdomen is suspicious. Unfortunately, the most common site of ischemic pain, the precordial substernal region, is identical with the incision for most cardiac repairs. Detection of ischemic pain in the preverbal child is more difficult, but if suspected, closer monitoring at the ECG, ST segments, and echo for wall motion abnormalities is indicated. Failure to recognize and treat ischemic cardiac pain in children may result in significant morbidity and mortality.

Having excluded the most common cause of cardiac pain in adults, it is interesting to review the unusual sources of cardiac pain for the child. Structural abnormalities such as idiopathic hypertropic subaortic stenosis (IHSS) only rarely produce pain in children. Of children who experienced sudden death from IHSS, only 7% reported any previous symptoms of chest pain.[73] Aortic stenosis, which is associated with chest pain in adults, does not appear to produce pain in children.[71] Mitral valve prolapse, which has a prevalence of 5% to 22% in female children, is a potential source of pain.[71] Vague nonexertional chest pain is concurrent with mitral valve prolapse in children and is the presenting complaint in about 8% to 18% of these children.[74,75] The association of mitral valve prolapse with other structural abnormalities such as atrial septal defects makes this problem potentially challenging in the postoperative period.[76]

Other noncardiac sources of chest pain should not be ignored in the postoperative period. The chest evacuation tubes are potential sites of pain by a variety of different mechanisms. Receptors from the skin and deeper tissues produce sensations such as pressure, position, and temperature, which are often interpreted as pain. Movement of the tube or change in suction intensify the painful response. This pain mechanism is poorly understood. Studies do not demonstrate an advantage of narcotics compared to placebo for the control of discomfort related to chest tube removal.[77]

The gastrointestinal tract is another factor in the differential diagnosis of chest pain. Gastrointestinal symptoms may mimic thoracic pathology due to their location within the thorax or upper abdomen. Mesenteric arteritis is a classic postoperative pain syndrome after coarctation repair. Esophageal reflux, esophageal spasm, biliary spasm, and peptic ulcers are other gastrointestinal sources of postoperative pain.

Finally, psychogenic causes must also be considered. Conversion symptoms producing chest pain have been noted in children as young as 7 years of age.[72] Depression has been identified as a cause of chest pain in children as young as 6 years of age.[78]

THE BASICS OF PEDIATRIC PAIN MANAGEMENT

Anticipation

Assume that any event you (the caregiver) would perceive as painful in the awake state will hurt a child. Pain management instituted prior to the application of a painful stimulus may be even more effective. Prevention of pain is easier than treatment, so pain management must begin as soon as the cutting edge penetrates the skin. The work by Wall supports this approach.[79] He has identified that in the absence of analgesia, pain can produce a reflex arc in the C-pain fibers.

Once this arc is initiated, it takes more analgesics to break it than it would have to prevent it.

Assessment and Reassessment

Regular reassessment of the problem and assessment of patient response to the therapy is the foundation of an effective medical therapeutic regimen. Monitoring of pain control methods is essential. Appropriate pain assessment in the pediatric patient is a difficult but not insurmountable task. The key is to select an assessment tool appropriate for the child's age and cognitive or developmental level. Exposure to pain evaluation tools should be initiated before the painful stimulus whenever possible. At this time, the child is not distracted by pain or any of the other discomforting events of the recovery phase. Practice with the pain assessment scale in a calm, pain-free setting helps the child label the pain when the experience does occur. Appropriateness of the selected measurement tool for an individual child can also be evaluated. An alternative method can be selected and prepared if the primary tool is ineffectual.

Pain assessment tools are necessarily based on behavioral and physiologic changes in young infants, toddlers, and nonverbal children of all ages. The operational pain scoring system (OPS) integrates both behavioral and physiologic variables. Behaviors associated with pain in the neonate include facial expressions, vocalizations, position of the extremities, and response to comfort.[80] The Children's Hospital of Eastern Ontario Pain Scale (CHEOPS) scoring system is effective in young children (1–7 years).[81] CHEOPS, designed for use in the immediate postoperative period in children, utilizes behavioral assessment. These measurement tools are limited, because they indicate the presence or absence of pain more reliably than its severity or location.[80] These scales can be enhanced by combination with a self-report method in children who are older than 3 years.

The ability to describe, compare, and relate pain to external events is a major developmental stage for the child. When this is possible, interactive pain assessment methods are more reliable and scientifically valid. Scaling systems based on pictures, colors, or poker chips are best for preschool children; visual and linear analog scales may be used with school-aged children.[82] These methods attempt to quantify an inherently subjective and probably nonlinear experience. Quantification is necessary for the scientific study of pain and its treatment. Objective scoring systems allow comparison between patients, or as a function of time and therapy in a single patient. Our primary pain assessment tool is the "Oucher."[83] This pictorial relative scale can be effectively used by children aged 3 years or older (see Figure 5–1). The accompanying numerical linear analog scale is helpful in older children.

The hallmark of adult pain assessment tools is the McGill pain questionnaire.[84] The original questionnaire is limited by its length and by its use of complex descriptive vocabulary, which may not be

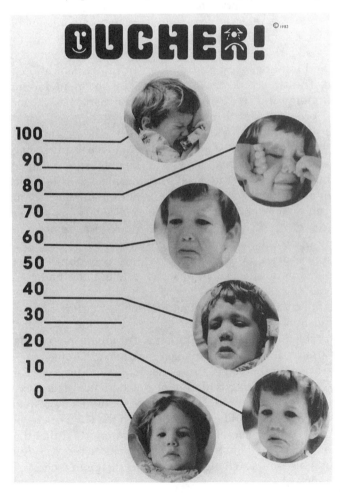

FIGURE 5–1. Pain scoring system used in children older than 3 years of age. (*The Oucher, Developed and copyrighted by Judith E. Beyer, RN., Ph.D., 1983. Reprinted with permission.*)

understood by even educated adults. For example, "lancinating" is an adjective that is not commonly recognized. Few patients are motivated to complete several pages of information as a prerequisite to obtaining analgesic medication. This comprehensive scoring system has been adapted for use in adolescence.[85] Tessler et al. have identified and categorized words that children typically use to describe pain. Words such as "scratch" and "pinch" describe minimal pain. "Aching" and "hurting" denote intermediate levels of pain. Moderate pain is "tearing" and "sharp." Death imagery such as "killing" and "shooting" is reserved for the most severe pain imaginable.[85]

A major confounding variable in the assessment and management of pediatric pain is the role of the parents. Parental opinions, biases, and attitudes may lead to over- or undermedication of their children. The caregivers may fear parental involvement. It diminishes their autonomy and sense of control and can disrupt established routine and protocol. Health professionals may be uncomfortable with the external scrutiny provided by the family. The parents, however, usually know the child best and can be a valuable resource in optimal pain therapy. Parental involvement in the child's pain management is best initiated prior to the onset of pain, integral with the learning of a pain assessment tool. The introduction of an objective measure of pain can establish rapport and serve to raise questions and resolve differences of opinion in a controlled, noncritical setting. This anticipatory approach can minimize postoperative problems and the awkwardness of a third party in the physician– or nurse–patient relationship. Parents can also be instructed about the nature of pain management.

Scientific data suggest several reasonable starting points, which may need minor adjustments or major redirection as a function of unpredictable individual characteristics. Although the parents' input may be useful, it also must be taken in context. Parents may be less effective at rating their child's response to a scientific procedure than they are at summarizing a more global experience. The parents' response to a specific procedural stimulus is more likely to reflect the parents' own feelings and expectations than the child's behavior during the procedure.[86] Therefore, we feel it is important that the child, nurse, and parent evaluate the baseline pain at rest in addition to procedural discomfort (change in position, suctioning, chest physical therapy, etc.).

Recent criticism of pediatric pain scoring systems suggests that they do not accurately assess the child's pain but reflect the cognitive and developmental stage of the child. One study examined the pain scoring system after a minor limited acute incident (blood drawing).[86]

Retrospective use of pain scoring systems in children were inaccurate. In this setting, children's reports of pain at the end of the procedure did not correlate with pain behavior observed during the procedure. However, utilization of pain scoring methods in the course of current and continuous pain such as during the postoperative period is still valid.

There is no single scoring system that can be utilized for every patient, nor has one tool been identified as superior in all situations. Familiarity with and regular use of a pain assessment tool is more important than the specific method. Utilization and documentation of pain scores at frequent intervals (every 1–4 hours) provides feedback to the caregivers. Pain monitoring allows assessment of the efficacy of a pain management strategy and response to any necessary modifications. The pain assessment tool needs to be appropriate for the age of the patient, appropriate to the type of pain being evaluated, appealing and attractive to use, easy to use and explain, valid, and reliable.

Duration

The duration of pain following cardiac surgery in adults has been shown to be at least 4 days and may be 6 days or greater.[87] The duration of pain in children following cardiac surgery has never been closely examined. The study of Beyer et al., on postoperative cardiac pain in children, assumed that the significant interval for postoperative pain is the first 3 postoperative days.[4] Indeed, in their study, children did not receive narcotics after the third day. That study's conclusions inferred that children experience postoperative pain as intensely as adults do but for a shorter period. No assessment of the presence or severity of pain was performed during this study. Our clinical and experimental experience indicate that adequate pain control in children undergoing cardiac surgery, that is, pain scores of less than 3/10, maintained through the first 48 hours postoperatively facilitate transition to non-narcotic agents on the third postoperative day.

PAIN MANAGEMENT APPROACHES

Two approaches to pediatric pain management are possible. Anticipatory protocols focus on the prevention of pain and attempt to avoid the experience of pain. A more conservative approach is to withhold therapy until pain is established.

Anticipatory

Recent investigations have begun to examine the neural mechanisms responsible for the development of pain. Pain pathways have been demonstrated in association with C-fibers in the spinal cord. Stimulation of these pathways continues during general anesthesia.[88] This spinal bombardment by pain afferent impulses initiates a prolonged and widespread increase in reflex excitability. This response is especially intense and prolonged if the stimulus comes from deep tissues rather than skin alone. Once these changes in cord excitability are established, it requires a very substantial narcotic dose to suppress the hyperexcitable state. The dose of narcotic required to prevent C-fiber excitability changes in the spinal cord is an order of magnitude lower than that required to suppress the changes in C-fiber excitability once they have occurred. This data favors prevention of pain in preference to symptomatic treatment. When a symptomatic approach is taken to pain management, the existence of pain is frequently determined retrospectively.[89] After the administration of an analgesic, an increase in the child's activity and movement and improvement in behavior, sleeping, and eating patterns verifies the prior existence of pain.

Responsive

The rates and sites of narcotic metabolism and elimination may vary with patient age. Onset and duration of action are dependent on lipid solubility and protein binding, which also change as a function of age, as even the preterm infant handles narcotics differently than the term neonate.[90] Table 5–1 depicts the available pharmacokinetic information by age group for commonly used opiods. Neonates demonstrate an increased susceptibility to the respiratory depressant effects of the opioids. Incomplete formation of the blood–brain barrier allows increased penetration of nonlipophilic narcotics such as morphine. There is also a relative increase in the proportion of Mu-2 receptors in the neonate.[90] The Mu-2 receptors are responsible for respiratory depression. It would seem logical to conclude that the neonate needs a smaller dose at a longer interval, but this is not true for all opiates. In neonates and children the increase in α-lipoproteins in the blood has the effect of increasing the apparent volume of distribution for highly lipid soluble drugs, thus, more drug might be necessary to produce the same effect.

However, because of decreased protein binding in the neonate, more free drug may be available. The summation of these effects in the neonate results in drug doses similar to those in older children. Clearance and metabolism may be altered by the maturing excretory systems, so the duration of action is commonly extended (see Table 5–1).

PAIN MANAGEMENT OPTIONS

The literature contains few reports concerning management of postoperative pain following pediatric cardiac or thoracic surgery.

P.R.N.

Pro re nata narcotics by intramuscular or intravenous intermittent bolus have been the standard of care for many years.[91] All too often, however, "as needed" is interpreted to mean "as little as possible and as infrequently as possible." When given alternatives, nurses may frequently choose the least potent analgesic. Children will frequently tolerate discomfort rather than receive an intramuscular injection for analgesia. P.r.n. narcotic administration is time-consuming and requires that pain precede analgesia.

Continuous Infusion

This method of delivering narcotics is effective and time efficient. Continuous infusion methods eliminate the peaks and troughs of analgesic delivery and minimize side effects. Following congenital heart surgery, a mean morphine dose between 10 to 30 μg/kg/hr appears necessary for pain control with a minimum analgesic blood level of 12 ng/mL.[92]

In neonates at risk for a pulmonary vascular hypertensive crisis, a routine postoperative continuous narcotic (fentanyl or sufentanil) infusion is recommended for 48 hours. The goals are to provide analgesia and blunt the stress response. Plasma fentanyl concentrations >20 ng/mL are required during surgery to achieve these effects.[93] Our treatment protocol for these high-risk neonates includes a fentanyl loading dose ≥35 mcg/kg followed by a continuous infusion at 0.3 mcg/kg/min. Koren et al. have demonstrated that the pharmacokinetic properties of fentanyl may change in children following cardiac surgery, so that the child may need additional bolus doses to maintain a steady state concentration.[94] Acute tolerance can occur when fentanyl is used at this dosage for sedation and analgesia. Anand has reported improved outcome in neonates who were maintained postoperatively on a continuous narcotic infusion.[64,65,68] He reported sufentanil infusion rates at 2 to 4 mcg/kg/hr and fentanyl infusion rates at 8 to 15 mcg/kg/hr.[68]

PATIENT-CONTROLLED ANALGESIA

Success with patient-controlled analgesia (PCA) has been reported in children undergoing thoracic surgery and in children as young as 5 years of age.[95] We believe that any child who can differentiate painful stimuli on a pain scoring system and can play video games is a candidate for PCA. To evaluate his or her ability to differentiate painful stimuli, ask the child to rate real life situations, such as mosquito bite, bee sting, falling off a bicycle, and the like. The ability to differentiate is more important than the specific number they assign. A patient-controlled analgesic method has significant physiologic and psychologic advantages.[96] PCA enhances patients' feelings of well-being, restores self-confidence, and replaces helplessness with a sense of control. Patients do not have a significant delay between the request for and delivery of analgesic medication.[96] The total analgesic dose delivered is often lower in PCA patients when compared to similar patients managed with a traditional intravenous regimen.[97] Lange et al., found that in thoracotomy patients, PCA was associated with a lower incidence of postoperative fever and pulmonary complications than was intramuscular delivery.[97]

Preoperative education and preparation are essential to the optimal use of PCA[98] even more for a child than for an adult. When a child is in pain, the ability to understand the workings of the machine is hampered by the cognitive state of development. Equipment costs are easily balanced by the benefits of improved nursing efficiency. In patients too young to use PCA, parent- or nurse-assisted PCA is an option. In parent-assisted PCA, the parent helps the child to identify and evaluate the pain. Parents are instructed not to push the PCA button unless directly instructed by the child to do so. Nurse-controlled analgesia utilizes the PCA machine to deliver unit doses of narcotics. The ready availability of narcotics encourages the nurse to maintain patient comfort. The patient's pain control can be more

TABLE 5-2. PCA Dosing in Children

	Morphine	Meperidine	Hydromorphone	Fentanyl
Loading dose	0.05–0.15 mg/kg	0.5–1.5 mg/kg	15–30 µg/kg	1–2 µg/kg
Infusion rate	0.01–0.03 mg/kg/hr	0.1–0.3 mg/kg/hr	1.5–4.5 µg/kg/hr	0.1–0.3 µg/kg/hr
Demand dose	0.02–0.04 mg/kg	0.2–0.4 mg/kg	4–8 µg/kg	0.2–0.4 µg/kg
4-hour limit	0.25–0.4 mg/kg	2.5–4.0 mg/kg	0.03–0.06 mg/kg	3–6 µg/kg
Lockout time	8–15 min	8–15 min	10–15 min	5–10 min

readily titrated using the small frequent PCA morphine doses (0.025–0.05 mg/kg) instead of standard fixed bolus doses (0.1 mg/kg) at longer intervals. In nurse-controlled analgesia, the nurse carries the patient control button. Administration of medication is achieved by plugging in the button and pushing it. The significant time saving and convenience of not having to go to the narcotic cabinet facilitates the nurse's ability to make the child comfortable.

In the immediate postoperative period, the patient may be too sleepy to use PCA appropriately. When PCA alone is attempted, it may result in higher pain intensity scores in the early postoperative period.[99] During this interval comfort should probably be achieved through a long-acting intraoperative analgesic, a continuous narcotic infusion, or nurse-administered medication.

PCA is initiated with a loading dose, which may be given during the surgical procedure, or in the Intensive Care Unit or recovery room. The incremental dose is programmed, and a lockout interval (8–12 minutes) is set during which the patient cannot receive another dose. The lockout interval allows the incremental dose to take effect before delivering a subsequent dose. Finally, a 4-hour total dose limit is set (0.25–0.5 mg/kg morphine). One variation of this system is labeled PCA Plus, which combines a low dose continuous narcotic infusion (morphine 10–40 µg/kg/hr) with the availability of a slightly decreased (morphine 0.018–0.045 mg/kg) incremental demand dose. The advantages of PCA Plus in children are less sedation and lower pain scores.[100] The continuous infusion can be discontinued when the patient's PCA incremental demand frequency decreases. Table 5–2 suggests recommended dosing when narcotics other than morphine are utilized.

The side effects observed with PCA narcotics are similar to those that accompany other methods of administering these drugs. In the presence of continued narcotic demand, diphenhydramine (0.25–0.5 mg/kg) is prescribed for pruritus and metoclopramide (0.1–0.2 mg/kg) for nausea and vomiting. If the side effects and pain persist, change to a different narcotic may be effective. Meperidine is the primary alternative agent, but hydromorphone may also be utilized.

SPINAL (EPIDURAL OR SUBARACHNOID) ANALGESIC TECHNIQUES

Intraspinal analgesia with either local anesthetics or opiates offers the best quality pain control. Various studies in adults undergoing thoracic surgery show that postoperative epidural or subarachnoid opioids improve analgesic quality, reduce the stress response, decrease total narcotic dose, or improve pulmonary function when compared to intravenous opioids or intercostal nerve blocks.[101–104]

Epidural morphine is also effective in children for pain control after thoracic or cardiac surgery. It is technically difficult and unnecessary to perform a thoracic epidural injection in small children to control thoracic pain, because injection of water soluble opiates through the caudal canal is safe and effective.[105] Long, small bore catheters (24 gauge) may be inserted into the thoracic region from the caudal inlet in infants for delivery of local anesthetic drugs or lipid soluble opiates.[106] In most children older than 3 years, it is difficult to advance long catheters to the thoracic region.

Several modifiers of spinal analgesic pharmacology have been reported. The duration of intrathecal analgesia was extended by mixing the drug with normal saline instead of dextrose.[107] The hypobaric mixture potentially facilitates spread of the drug to the dermatomes responsible for the pain. The choice of opioid determines the duration of analgesia and the potential for distant spread of analgesic effects (see Chapter 1).

The duration of analgesia from bolus doses of epidural morphine in children varies, with durations of 4 hours to greater than 24 hours reported. The mean duration we have observed as 10 hours. The recommended bolus dose in children ranges from 0.05 to 0.10 mg/kg. Our protocol uses 0.075 mg/kg diluted to a volume of 10 ml of preservative-free saline if the morphine dose is greater than 1 mg, or 5 ml of preservative-free saline if the morphine dose is less than 1 mg. Investigating the effects of repeated epidural morphine administration in children, Krane et al., found no prolongation of effect or acute tolerance, but the numbers of patients were relatively small.[108]

Continuous epidural infusion techniques decrease the number of narcotic molecules in the CSF at any one time, allowing spinal cord and epidural fat to serve as drug reservoirs. Saturation of the peridural fat could result in rostral spread of even lipophilic drugs such as fentanyl.[109] We initiate continuous epidural morphine infusions in children with a bolus of 0.04 mg/kg followed by a continuous infusion of 0.125 mcg/kg/min. The morphine is diluted as in the previous intermittent bolus group. Those patients who receive the morphine diluted in 5 ml receive a constant infusion at 0.5 ml/hr, while the other group receives an infusion at 1 ml/hr. Local anesthetic continuous infusions epidural have also been found effective.

Continuous epidural infusions in pediatric patients are facilitated by the availability of fine small bore (24 gauge) catheters. These small epidural catheters have a lower failure rate when they are continuously infused as compared to intermittent boluses of medications.[123] A practical concern in small children is the optimal method for securing these catheters. The life expectancy of the catheter increases if it courses to the patient's side as opposed to up the back. Hygiene and sterility are concerns unique to caudally placed epidural catheters. We utilize a double dressing technique. One is placed caudad to the epidural catheter and one cephalad to it to sandwich the epidural catheter inside, making it possible to keep the insertion site clean even if the child defecates.

Combinations of local anesthetics and epidural narcotics are also effective. The dose of local anesthetic is calculated considering the location of the tip of the catheter with Takasaki's formula (0.056 ml/kg/segment = the volume of local anesthetic).[110] Bupivacaine, 0.0625% to 0.1%, can be selected. Uptake from the epidural space is rapid and it is important to remember that the toxic dose of bupivacaine in children is approximately 3 mg/kg (or 0.25 mg/kg/hr).[111] The catheter should be checked at regular intervals to ensure that it has not migrated into the subarachnoid or intravenous space. If the catheter is close to the spinal dermatome responsible for the pain stimulus, fentanyl may be added to deliver a dose of 0.5 to 2 mcg/kg/hr. Fentanyl has been used epidurally as a sole analgesic agent, although its mechanism of action is controversial.[112] Glass et al. concluded that the analgesic effects of epidural fentanyl are primarily mediated by systemic absorption.[113] Other epidural opiates, such as sufentanil, methadone, hydromorphone, diamorphine, and meperidine, have been given infrequently,[114,115,116] (see Table 5–3).

Many studies examining the use of spinally administered analgesics have reported the need for supplemental systemic narcotics. The basis for this practice can be derived from an examination of the pathways used to transmit the nociceptive information. Epidural opiates are known to work locally in the spinal cord by binding to the

TABLE 5–3. Epidural Opiate Dosing

Drug	Liquid Solubility	Bolus (μg/kg)	Infusion (μg/kg/hr)
Methadone	116	150	20
Alfentanil	126	15	
Sufentanil	1778	0.75	
Fentanyl	813	1.5	0.2–0.7
Hydromorphone			1
Morphine	1.4	0.4	4–8

opiate receptors in the substantia gelatinosa. Pain is transmitted along a variety of pathways, but A-delta fibers and C-fibers are responsible for much of its transmission. The continuous pain produced by damage to visceral tissues is transmitted along C-fibers, whereas the sharp pain of an incision is transmitted along A-delta fibers. C-fibers from the periphery terminate in the substantia gelatinosa in association with opiate receptors. In contrast, A-delta fibers usually transmit their information to the brain without opioid receptor modulation of spinal synapses. Therefore, systemic opioids may be necessary to address the pain transmitted along A-delta fibers, although this increases the incidence of opiate side effects.

All routes of administration of narcotics carry the risk of respiratory depression. The possibility of delayed respiratory depression poses a unique disadvantage to intraspinal narcotics. Although intrathecal opiates (morphine 0.02 mg/kg) provide effective long-term analgesia in children, the incidence of side effects, particularly late respiratory depression, has limited their clinical usefulness in treatment of acute pain.[117] In contrast, not only are epidural narcotics very effective in children, but also reports of early or late respiratory depression are uncommon.[118] The clinical appearance of respiratory depression following spinal narcotics in children is similar to that seen in adults. Usually there is increased sedation and a decrease in tidal volume that can occur without a decrease in respiratory rate. Monitoring these patients with simple apnea (chest wall impedance) monitors is therefore inadequate. A recent comprehensive review of spinal narcotics in pediatrics produced several clinical recommendations.[119] The period of increased risk for late respiratory depression was 8 to 10 hours after opiate injection. Only children who had received intrathecal morphine required naloxone reversal of clinically significant respiratory depression. It is important to note that respiratory depression has been reported as early as 3.5 hours after epidural morphine injection in children.[118]

Monitoring for delayed respiratory depression is rarely an issue following cardiac surgery, because intensive care monitoring and nursing are necessary. However, children undergoing thoracic procedures may not require intensive care monitoring. Standards of practice for children receiving spinal narcotics vary. Many centers have become familiar enough with spinal narcotics that patients receive routine postoperative nursing care without special monitoring, while other institutions require that these children receive continuous cardiorespiratory monitoring. The conservative approach is probably safest when initiating a new service. Respiratory depression does not appear to be a problem more than 8 hours after a bolus dose or more than 8 hours after initiating a constant rate of a continuous infusion. The greatest risk for respiratory depression occurs when supplemental intravenous narcotics are given in addition to epidural opiates. If late respiratory depression is the primary concern, using epidural local anesthetics, instead of opiates, avoids this problem as well as the minimal $PaCO_2$ elevation reported in adults.[103] Combinations of opioids and local anesthetics represent another possibility as this would permit a reduction in the dose of opioid administered.

Minor side effects (e.g., nausea and vomiting, pruritus, and urinary retention) seen with intravenous opioid analgesics also occur with epidurally administered opioids. A 1990 review of pediatric epidural opioids reported incidences of urinary retention, nausea and vomiting, and pruritus as 27%, 33% to 56%, and 22% to 57%, respectively. The incidence of side effects (vomiting and pruritus) is greatest after the first dose.[108] Vomiting occurs more often in patients who are fed early after surgery. One report describes dysphoria in a child following epidural morphine.[119]

Various methods have been proposed to minimize the side effects of spinal opiates. Concurrent administration of low-dose naloxone intravenously or the addition of droperidol (2.5 mg/70 kg) or butorphanol (40 mcg/kg) to the epidural injection have been reported.[120,121] We administer nalbuphine (0.025–0.05 mg/kg) intravenously to control pruritus and nausea, believing that it is more effective and exhibits fewer side effects than intravenous metoclopramide or diphenhydramine.

From 1986 to 1990, we routinely administered epidural morphine at the end of cardiac surgery after confirming heparin neutralization and assuming that clinical signs of a coagulopathy were absent. The rationale for this practice was to maximize the postoperative duration of a single epidural opiate injection.[86] Earlier administration of the first dose of spinal narcotics may be desirable, as Vanstrum et al. found a 35% reduction in the need for vasodilator therapy during cardiopulmonary bypass when intrathecal morphine was administered before incision.[122] Our current protocol has been modified to reflect this information.[123] Following induction of general anesthesia, attainment of intravenous access, and endotracheal intubation, the child is turned to the lateral decubitus position for placement of an epidural catheter via the caudal canal. The catheter is then aspirated and preservative-free morphine in saline is injected as described earlier. The child is then returned to the supine position, and additional invasive monitoring catheters are inserted. The time interval from the initial dosing of the epidural catheter to the onset of surgery is approximately 15 to 30 minutes, which allows for onset of the epidural morphine before incision. Using this approach, the beneficial effects we have observed include reduced general anesthetic requirements, which facilitates early postoperative extubation without sacrificing analgesia. Another advantage of intraoperative epidural morphine is that it is not subject to uptake by the membrane oxygenator during cardiopulmonary bypass.[124,125]

Epidural narcotics have been given to children as a single bolus injection, through a catheter by intermittent bolus injections, by continuous infusion, and by PCA.[102,106,124,126,127] Unfortunately, there is no comparative study of these techniques. However, adult data suggest that epidural PCA might be the best approach in children old enough to understand and use this modality effectively.[127–129]

ALTERNATIVE ROUTES OF NARCOTIC DELIVERY

There are relatively noninvasive alternatives to parenteral or spinal opiates. Some of these methods are inadequate for the control of acute postoperative pain, but may be appropriate later in the course of recovery. Oral medications have limited application in the immediate postoperative period due to the intensity of the pain and to the effects of surgery and anesthesia on gastric and intestinal motility.

The sublingual route has several advantages. Uptake from the buccal mucosa is more rapid and reliable than from the gastric mucosa, and normal gastrointestinal function is not required. Sublingual buprenorphine produces analgesia comparable to meperidine PCA.[130] Inadvertent swallowing of the medication does not cause overdose because of high first pass hepatic metabolism. In pediatric patients a high incidence of sedation and nausea limits buprenorphine use. Transmucosal fentanyl citrate (fentanyl lollipop) is the simplest drug to administer and has been used for sedation and analgesia.

Rectal administration of sedatives and antipyretics is a common pediatric practice. Rectal suppositories of hydromorphone and methadone are also available. Uptake from the rectal mucosa is rapid but may be limited by rectal contents or by reflex evacuation of the rectum. A sustained release rectal morphine formulation frequently does not provide complete pain relief, but can be used to provide baseline opiate coverage for other intermittent on-demand techniques.[131]

Transdermal delivery of medications such as fentanyl presents an interesting alternative. Fentanyl patches provide a sustained release of up to 100 mcg/hr. The major disadvantage is the 2-hour onset time. This technique should not be used to achieve control of acute pain but is satisfactory for maintenance of analgesia. An intravenous fentanyl bolus dose is necessary to establish therapeutic blood levels.[132] Transdermal fentanyl is available in four mixed dosage forms. Unfortunately these patches should not be trimmed or modified because significant changes in drug delivery can result. When fluid restriction is a primary concern, the patch can be used to maintain an effective plasma fentanyl level without additional intravenous fluid. A 100 mcg/hr patch could provide a steady delivery of 0.16 mcg/kg/min in a 10 kg patient.

NON-NARCOTIC ANALGESIC METHODS

Opiates are not universally required for the control of pain. In some cases, alternative medications are adequate or even indicated. Musculoskeletal pains often respond better to non-steroidal anti-inflammatory drugs (NSAIDs), such as acetaminophen or ibuprofen, than to opioids. The introduction of a parenteral NSAID (ketorolac 0.5–1 mg/kg) allows this form of treatment to begin earlier. Ketorolac can be given intravenously or intramuscularly.[133,134] IM medications are not recommended for control of postoperative pain in children unless the intravenous or oral routes are unavailable. When given intravenously, the dose should be infused over a 10-minute period to avoid pain at the site of installation. This drug is most effective when a loading dose of 1 mg/kg is given followed by 0.5 mg/kg every 6 hours around the clock. The potential for this drug to produce platelet dysfunction has generated some concern in cardiothoracic surgery. The dysfunction reverses on drug discontinuation and appears to have minimal clinical significance in most cases. Sternotomy has been associated with a significant incidence of upper rib fractures.[135] NSAIDs, in addition to opioids, should be considered for pain control in such cases or when rib resection is performed.

Acetaminophen is useful in combination with narcotics. The acetaminophen potentiates analgesia without increasing the incidence of side effects. Usually, either a NSAID or acetaminophen is utilized. If the patient is febrile, however, the medications may be alternated so that an antipyretic medication is given as frequently as possible. This may also enhance the analgesic potential.

The utility of local anesthetics was introduced in the section on spinal analgesia. Local anesthetics can be deposited in many locations other than the epidural space. Intercostal nerve blocks have been recognized for a long time for their ability to produce analgesia. There is no doubt that they are effective. The major limitation of intercostal blocks in children is the relatively short duration, rarely exceeding 8 hours. Few awake children cooperate with repetition of the nerve blocks. Placement of an intercostal catheter has been reported to extend the duration of nerve block. The catheter is placed near the angle of the rib and then into the intercostal space one level below the one opened for surgery. Injections through the catheter can then be administered as an intermittent bolus or infused continuously.[136] A variation of the intercostal approach is the use of intrapleural local anesthetics to provide postoperative analgesia. The quality of analgesia can be very good, but the technique is limited by the frequent technical difficulties of catheter placement and maintenance.[137,138]

Other classes of drugs also have been recognized for their abilities to produce analgesia. Analgesia is a well-known side effect of several classes of antihypertensives. Alpha-2 agonists, such as clonidine, have been found to be particularly effective when administered either epidurally or intravenously to adults.[139,140] The postulated mechanism is inhibition of substance P release. Clonidine epidural analgesia begins within 20 minutes and lasts for 5 hours. Blood pressure reduction may begin within the first hour. Bradycardia also has been observed when this drug is administered epidurally. In pediatric patients, clonidine serves as an effective oral adjunct to many analgesic regimens. A dose of 3 to 5 mcg/kg every 8 hours enhances analgesia and induces mild sedation. Clonidine is a potent antihypertensive agent in adults, but the effects on blood pressure in children appear to be minimal. We have observed bradycardia as the only problematic side effect. Beta receptor blockers and calcium channel blockers have also been reported to enhance analgesic effects of narcotics. Calcium channel blockers may produce this effect by inhibition of calcium release from nociceptive nerves in the periphery.[141]

Nonpharmacologic techniques for pain modulation are also available. Parental presence, massage, and relaxation and distraction techniques are effective.[142,143] Psychological support in the form of behavior modification therapy may improve patient comfort.[144] These methods should be used in addition to pharmacologic agents rather than as a replacement for drug therapy. Transcutaneous electrical nerve stimulation may also be useful in children when incisional pain lasts longer than expected.[145]

Chest tube pain is also significant for patients who have undergone cardiac or thoracic surgery. This pain proves difficult to treat. An adult study found morphine to be no better than placebo in the relief of discomfort during chest tube removal.[78] A proposed mechanism of pain transmission with this procedure involves proprioceptive impulses, which are interpreted by the brain as pain. This is a plausible explanation because narcotics have no effect on proprioceptive fibers. The fibers responsible for proprioception are closely associated with those responsible for temperature sensation. We recommend the use of ice to reduce sensitivity to chest tube removal. At first the skin is insulated by wrapping the ice pack in several layers of cloth. The layers are gradually removed until the ice is sitting directly on the skin in close proximity to the chest tube insertion site. Infiltration of the insertion site with local anesthetic is a possible alternative, however, this procedure is inherently painful. The application of Eutectic Mixture of Local Anesthetics (EMLA) cream or drug delivery by iontophoresis are potential options. Iontophoresis of local anesthetic has been used in children with renal disease to facilitate painless shunt access. These methods have not been tested for chest tube procedures but are potentially beneficial. If EMLA cream is used, it should be placed over the chest tube site and covered by an occlusive dressing for 90 minutes before attempting manipulation of the chest tube.

SEDATION AS A COMPONENT OF PAIN MANAGEMENT

The experience of pain is not an isolated event. Pain or anticipation of pain is a significant source of anxiety. An increased level of anxiety produces autonomic arousal; autonomic arousal then increases muscular tone and increases pain.[146] This process constitutes a vicious cycle. Benzodiazepines have been shown to reduce pain by decreasing autonomic arousal and interrupting the self-perpetuating cycle. A classic study demonstrated a reduction in analgesic requirements through lessening of anxiety. Patients who were given in-depth, detailed prospective information about what to expect during their hospital course required half as much analgesics as those who were not educated about anticipated events.[147] The educational process is important, and the child who has the ability to grasp even simple concepts should have the preoperative experience explained in understandable terms.

An ideal sedative agent does not exist. All sedatives exhibit tolerance if given for a long enough period. Similar to analgesic regimens, the merits of intermittent bolus techniques as compared to continuous infusion techniques are commonly debated. Tolerance appears to occur more readily with continuous infusion (Figure 5–2) owing in part to inappropriate management. In clinical practice, an infusion rate is often preselected and maintained unless an increased dose is necessary, thus eliminating a major advantage to continuous infusion. We recommend frequent attempts to decrease the infusion level to the lowest possible continuous baseline dose (Figure 5–3), combined with increasing the infusion rate. The continuous baseline infusion rate is further decreased during sleep. When tolerance develops, the infusion rate may be increased, but this increases the incidence of side effects and withdrawal reactions. Many different drugs possess sedative properties (Figure 5–4). Narcotics are frequently utilized, but in the absence of pain these drugs are a poor choice for sedation. In the presence of pain, however, excellent analgesics may be impaired by inadequate sedation. The side effects of opiates are more pronounced when they are used as sedative agents. Tolerance, dependence, and addiction then become common problems. Dependence and addiction are seldom observed when narcotics are used for control of acute pain, but we have observed that depen-

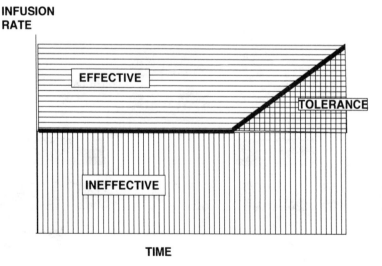

FIGURE 5–2. Keeping the infusion rate of sedative agents constant promotes the development of tolerance.

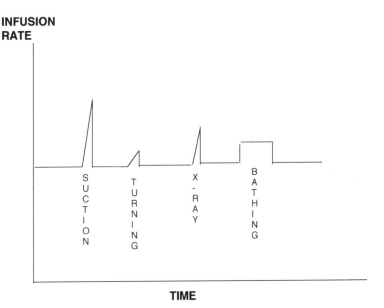

FIGURE 5–3. Adjusting infusion to the clinical situation limits the onset of tolerance.

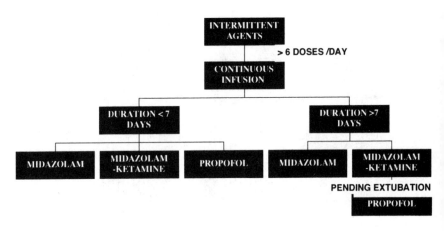

FIGURE 5–4. Algorithm for sedation in children during the postoperative period.

dence readily occurs when they are used for sedation alone. Physical dependence has been reported to occur after 5 days of narcotic sedation.[148-151]

Another drug with both intense analgesic and sedative properties is ketamine. Absence of respiratory depression and maintenance of myocardial function and vascular resistance are additional advantages. In adults, one study found ketamine could be used as the sole agent to provide sedation and analgesia, but another group of investigators could not reproduce these results without adding morphine.[152,153] Ketamine has been used effectively in the pediatric intensive care unit to provide sedation and analgesia.[154,155] There is a potential for negative psychotropic experiences related to ketamine use, although the risk of such occurrences appears to be greater in adults.

We prefer to combine ketamine infusion with low-dose midazolam continuous infusions. Sedation is adequate with this technique, and there is minimal need for supplemental narcotics after the first two postoperative days. Our infusion protocol uses a midazolam bolus (0.25 mg/kg) followed by a continuous infusion (0.4–4 mcg/kg/min) and a ketamine bolus (0.5 mg/kg) followed by a continuous infusion (10–70 mcg/kg/min). This protocol offers two distinct advantages over narcotic based sedation protocols: the ability to maintain spontaneous respirations and the ability to utilize the alimentary tract for nutrition. When high-infusion rates are maintained for prolonged periods, myoclonic movements frequently occur. These movements may persist as long as 1 month following ketamine therapy, but do spontaneously and gradually resolve. Increased oropharyngeal secretions uncommonly occur when ketamine is given by continuous infusion at low doses. Excessive secretions are easily controlled with glycopyrrolate.

Benzodiazepines possess many properties of a theoretically ideal sedative. Anxiolysis and sedation are the primary therapeutic effects. While not possessing intrinsic analgesic characteristics, benzodiazepines may enhance the analgesia produced by opiates. Respiratory or cardiovascular depression can occur, but are less of a problem than with adults. The safety of these drugs has been improved by the clinical availability of a specific antagonist, flumazenil. The introduction of the relatively short-acting midazolam has expanded the clinical spectrum of benzodiazepines to include continuous infusion techniques. Midazolam is optimally administered by continuous infusion in the same doses previously described for use with a ketamine infusion. When the guidelines are followed, dependence is rare with

TABLE 5–4. Sedation is Rated Hourly at Rest and With Stimulation Using Both the Behavioral and Physiologic Scoring Systems

Sedation Flow Sheet

Behavioral Score

0 COMA	1 ASLEEP	2 DROWSY	3 CALM	4 AWAKE	5 WILD
Eyes closed	Eyes closed	Eyes open or closed	Eyes open	Alert	Anxious
No motion	Rare spon. motion	Moves '0–5' times/min.	Moves 5–10 times/min.	Active, moves >10 times/ min	Excess motion
No head motion	No head motion	No head motion	Minimal head motion	Slow head motion	Tosses head from side to side
No arm or leg motion	Minimal arm or leg motion	Moves arms or legs	Moves arms or legs	Moves arms and legs	Thrashes arms and legs
No reaction to stimulus	No reaction to mild stimulus	Eyes open with mild stimulus	Moves on command	Easy to control movements	No control of movements

Physiologic Score

	a	b	c
HR	<10%	Baseline	>10%
BP	<10%	Baseline	>10%
Resp.	<10%	Baseline	>10%
Pupil	small	midsize	large

Place a "P" beside score if patient is receiving muscle relaxant.

Time	Rest Sedation Score		Stimulated Sedation Score	
	Behav.	Physio.	Behav.	Physio.

midazolam infusion even after several weeks of continuous therapy and hemodynamic depression is minimal with midazolam in most patients.[156] Amnesia is potentially the most valuable effect of benzodiazepine administration. Suppressing memory of the entire intensive care experience exerts potential psychologic benefits for both the child and the family.

Propofol has been used to provide sedation and enhance narcotic analgesia. A number of papers have discussed this approach in adults following cardiac surgery.[157–159] Sedation is initiated by incremental boluses of 0.25 mg/kg until the child becomes appropriately sedated. Total bolus dose ranges from 0.5 to 3.0 mg/kg, then a continuous infusion is started at 50 mcg/kg/min. The infusion is titrated between 20 and 300 mcg/kg/min to maintain the desired level of sedation. When short-term sedation (less than 24 h) is needed, propofol offers the possible advantages over midazolam of earlier awakening and greater augmentation of morphine analgesia, although amnesia is not reliably produced. Limitations include tolerance, dependence, and hypotension. Propofol induces transient depression of myocardial contractility and more prolonged systemic vasodilation.[160] Propofol-induced hypotension usually responds readily to intravenous fluid replacement. Tolerance to propofol may develop rapidly, necessitating increases in the infusion rate. After approximately 7 days, even increasing the infusion does not deal with the tolerance. After approximately 4 days of continuous propofol infusion, gradual weaning may be required in order to avoid a withdrawal syndrome.[161] An additional concern with continuous infusion of propofol is the prevention of bacterial growth in the intralipid carrier solution. The drug is therefore meticulously prepared by the pharmacy.

It is important to differentiate analgesic and sedative requirements in children during the postoperative period and treat each problem with the appropriate medication. To facilitate sedative titration, we use the scoring system shown in Table 5–4. Instructions for manipulation of infusion dose are referenced to the sedation score, increasing or decreasing the infusion when specific criteria are met. This method discourages excessive sedation, and tolerance and side effects are minimized by maintaining the lowest infusion rate.

SUMMARY AND CONCLUSION

The optimal approach to pain is one that never allows pain to occur. This implies that effective pain relief should be initiated before a surgical procedure and continue throughout recovery (Figure 5–5). We

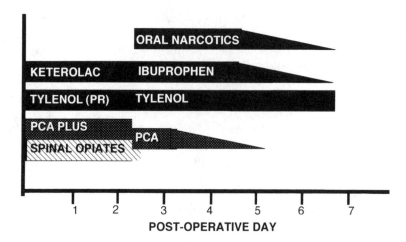

FIGURE 5–5. This figure demonstrates options for pediatric postoperative analgesic options. It depicts analgesic options which may be given on the various days. For example, on days 1 and 2 PCA Plus or spinal opiates may be used. Concurrently, acetaminophen and/or keterolac could be used on days 1 and 2. By day 2-1/2 the patient may be ready to go to oral narcotics, and changing to oral ibuprofen or acetaminophen makes sense. Additionally, if the child was using PCA Plus by day 2-1/2, the child should be able to use PCA without the continuous background infusion.

believe that caudal epidural morphine administered before the onset of pain provides optimal analgesia, supplementing this technique with small doses of intravenous morphine as needed. PCA Plus would be our second choice if the child is able to cooperate. Continuous infusion of a narcotic would be our next alternative. An age-appropriate pain assessment tool should be regularly used to assess the effectiveness of therapy and direct modifications of the pain management plan.

We conclude with J. A. Wildsmith's words of wisdom about the current status of pain management: "The message is clear: we have methods that are more than acceptable; what we must develop is the determination to utilize them effectively, safely, and in an appropriate manner."[162]

References

1. Gross S, Gardner G: Child pain: Treatment approaches. In Smith W, Mersky H, Gross S (eds): Pain: Meaning and Management, pp. 127–142. New York, SP Medical and Scientific Books, 1980

2. Swafford L, Allan D: Pain relief in the pediatric patient. Med Clin North Am 52(1):131–136, 1968
3. Beyer JE, DeGood DE, Ashley LC, Russell GA: Patterns of postoperative analgesic use with adults and children following cardiac surgery. Pain 17:71–81, 1983
4. Beyer JE, Ashley LC, Russell GA, DeGood DE: Pediatric pain after cardiac surgery: Pharmacologic management (research). Dimens Crit Care Nurs 3(6):326–334 (20 ref), 1984
5. Mather L, Mackie J: The incidence of postoperative pain in children. Pain 15:271–282, 1983
6. Schecter NL: The undertreatment of pain in children: An overview. Pediatr Clin North Am 36:781–794, 1989
7. Rasmussen G, Bell C, Snelling L, Gregus T, Glazer J: Analgesic dosing patterns in pediatric patients after open-heart surgery. Anesth Analg 74:s245, 1992
8. Anand KJS, Phil D, Hickey PR: Pain and its effects in the human neonate and fetus. N Engl J Med 317(21):1321–1329, 1987
9. Anand KJS, Phil D, Carr DB: The neuroanatomy, neurophysiology and neurochemistry of pain stress and analgesia in newborns and children. Pediatr Clin North Am 36:795–827, 1989
10. Moss IR, Conner H, Yee WFH, Iorio P, Scarpelli EM: Human B-endorphin-like immunoreactivity in the prenatal/neonatal period. J Pediatr 101:443–446, 1982
11. Lerman J, Robinson S, Willis MM, Gregory GA: Anesthetic requirements for halothane in young children 0–1 month and 1–6 months of age. Anesthesiology 59:421–424, 1983
12. Zeltzer LK, Fanurik D, LeBaron S: The cold pressor pain paradigm in children: Feasibility of an intervention model (Part II). Pain 37:305–313, 1989
13. LeBaron S, Zeltzer LK, Fanurik D: An investigation of the cold pressor pain in children (Part I). Pain 37:161–171, 1989
14. Beyer J, Aradine C: Content validity of an instrument to measure young children's perceptions on the intensity of their pain. J Pediatr Nurs 1(6):386–395, 1986
15. Lynn AM, Slattery JT: Morphine pharmacokinetics in early infancy. Anesthesiology 66:136–139, 1987
16. Bhat R, Chari G, Gulati A et al: Pharmacokinetics of a single dose of morphine in preterm infants during the first week of life. J Pediatr 117:477–481, 1990
17. Dahlstrom B, Bolme P, Feychting H et al: Morphine kinetics in children. Clin Pharmacol Ther 26(3):354–365, 1979
18. Glare PA, Walsh TD: Clinical pharmacokinetics of morphine. Ther Drug Monit 13(1):1–23, 1991
19. Hoskin PJ, Hanks GW, Aherne GW, Chapman D, Littleton P, Filshie J: The bioavailability and pharmacokinetics of morphine after intravenous, oral and buccal administration in healthy volunteers. Br J Clin Pharmacol 27(4):499–505, 1989
20. Dahlstrom B, Tamsen A, Paalzow L, Hartvig P: Patient-controlled analgesic therapy, Part IV: Pharmacokinetics and analgesic plasma concentrations of morphine. Clin Pharmacokinet 7(3):266–279, 1982
21. Garrett ER, Chandran VR: Pharmacokinetics of morphine and its sur-

rogates VI: Bioanalysis, solvolysis kinetics, solubility, pK'a values, and protein binding of buprenorphine. J Pharm Sci 74(5):515–524, 1985

22. Inturrisi CE, Colburn WA, Kaiko RF, Houde RW, Foley KM: Pharmacokinetics and pharmacodynamics of methadone in patients with chronic pain. Clin Pharmacol Ther 41(4):392–401, 1987

23. Meresaar U, Nilsson MI, Holmstrand J, Anggard E: Single dose pharmacokinetics and bioavailability of methadone in man studied with a stable isotope method. Eur J Clin Pharmacol 20(6):473–478, 1981

24. Schleimer R, Benjamini E, Eisele J, Henderson G: Pharmacokinetics of fentanyl as determined by radioimmunoassay. Clin Pharmacol Ther 23(2):188–194, 1978

25. Greeley WJ, de Bruijn NP, Davis DP: Sufentanil pharmacokinetics in pediatric cardiovascular patients. Anesth Analg 66(11):1067–1072, 1987

26. Chauvin M, Lebrault C, Levron JC, Duvaldestin P: Pharmacokinetics of alfentanil in chronic renal failure. Anesth Analg 66(1):53–56, 1987

27. Koren G, Goresky G, Crean P, Klein J, MacLeod SM: Pediatric fentanyl dosing based on pharmacokinetics during cardiac surgery. Anesth Analg 63(6):577–582, 1984

28. Shafer A, Sung ML, White PF: Pharmacokinetics and pharmacodynamics of alfentanil infusions during general anesthesia. Anesth Analg 65(10):1021–1028, 1986

29. Koehntop DE, Rodman JH, Brundage DM, Hegland MG, Buckley JJ: Pharmacokinetics of fentanyl in neonates. Anesth Analg 65(3):227–232, 1986

30. Camu F, Gepts E, Rucquoi M, Heykants J: Pharmacokinetics of alfentanil in man. Anesth Analg 61(8):657–661, 1982

31. Bentley JB, Borel JD, Nenad RE Jr, Gillespie TJ: Age and fentanyl pharmacokinetics. Anesth Analg 61(12):968–971, 1982

32. Chauvin M, Ferrier C, Haberer JP, Spielvogel C, Lebrault C, Levron JC, Duvaldestin P: Sufentanil pharmacokinetics in patients with cirrhosis. Anesth Analg 68(1):1–4, 1989

33. Bovill JG, Sebel PS, Blackburn CL, Oei-Lim V, Heykants JJ: The pharmacokinetics of sufentanil in surgical patients. Anesthesiology 61(5): 502–506, 1984

34. Goresky GV, Koren G, Sabourin MA, Sale JP, Strunin L: The pharmacokinetics of alfentanil in children. Anesthesiology 67(5):654–659, 1987

35. Bovill JG, Sebel PS, Blackburn CL, Heykants J: The pharmacokinetics of alfentanil (R39209): A new opioid analgesic. Anesthesiology 57(6):439–443, 1982

36. Meisterlman C, Saint-Maurice C, Lepaul M, Levron JC, Loose JP, Mac Gee K: A comparison of alfentanil pharmacokinetics in children and adults. Anesthesiology 66(1):13–16, 1987

37. Hudson RJ, Bergstrom RG, Thomson IR, Sabourin MA, Rosenbloom M, Strunin L: Pharmacokinetics of sufentanil in patients undergoing abdominal aortic surgery. Anesthesiology 70(3):426–431, 1989

38. Hudson RJ, Thomson IR, Cannon JE, Friesen RM, Meatherall RC: Pharmacokinetics of fentanyl in patients undergoing abdominal aortic surgery. Anesthesiology 64(3):334–338, 1986

39. Guay J, Gaudreault P, Tang A, Goulet B, Varin F: Pharmacokinetics of sufentanil in normal children. Can J Anaesth 39(1):14–20, 1992

40. Roure P, Jean N, Leclerc AC, Cabanel N, Levron JC, Duvaldestin P: Pharmacokinetics of alfentanil in children undergoing surgery. Br J Anaesth 59(11):1437–1440, 1987
41. Matteo RS, Schwartz AE, Ornstein E, Young WL, Chang W: Pharmacokinetics of sufentanil in the elderly surgical patient. Can J Anaesth 37(8):852–856, 1990
42. Duthie DJ, McLaren AD, Nimmo WS: Pharmacokinetics of fentanyl during constant rate i.v. infusion for the relief of pain after surgery. Br J Anaesth 58(9):950–956, 1986
43. Chauvin M, Salbaing J, Perrin D, Levron JC, Viars P: Clinical assessment and plasma pharmacokinetics associated with intramuscular or extradural alfentanil. Br J Anaesth 57(9):886–891, 1985
44. Van Beem H, Van Peer A, Gasparini R, Woestenborghs R, Heykants J, Noorduin H, Van Egmond J, Crul J: Pharmacokinetics of alfentanil during and after a fixed rate infusion. Br J Anaesth 62(6):610–615, 1989
45. Singleton MA, Rosen JI, Fisher DM: Pharmacokinetics of fentanyl in the elderly. Br J Anaesth 60(6):619–622, 1988
46. Scott JC, Stanski DR: Decreased fentanyl and alfentanil dose requirements with age. A simultaneous pharmacokinetic and pharmacodynamic evaluation. J Pharmacol Exp Ther 240(1):159–166, 1987
47. Shafer SL, Varvel JR: Pharmacokinetics, pharmacodynamics and rational opioid selection. Anesthesiology 74:53–63, 1991
48. David PT, Cook DR, Stiller RL, Davin-Robinson KA: Pharmacodynamics and pharmacokinetics of high-dose sufentanil in infants and children undergoing cardiac surgery. Anesthesiology 66:203–208, 1987
49. Gauntlett IS, Fisher DM, Hertzka RE, Kuhis E, Spellman MJ, Rudolph C: Pharmacokinetics of fentanyl in neonatal humans and lambs: Effects of age. Anesthesiology 69:683–687, 1988
50. Gourlay GK, Wilson PR, Glynn CJ: Pharmacodynamics and pharmacokinetics of methadone during the perioperative period. Anesthesiology 57:458–467, 1982
51. Greeley WJ, de Bruijn NP: Changes in sufentanil pharmacokinetics within the neonatal period. Anesth Analg 67:86–90, 1988
52. Baillie SP, Bateman DN, Coates PE, Woodhouse KW: Age and the pharmacokinetics of morphine. Age Ageing 18:258–262, 1989
53. Mather LE: Clinical pharmacokinetics of fentanyl and its newer derivatives. Clin Pharmacokinet 8:422–446, 1983
54. Bower S, Hull CJ: Comparative pharmacokinetics of fentanyl and alfentanil. Br J Anaesth 54:871–877, 1982
55. Halliburton JR: The pharmacokinetics of fentanyl, sufentanil and alfentanil: A comparative review. AANA J 56(3):229–233, 1988
56. Lutz LJ, Lamer TJ: Management of postoperative pain: Review of current techniques and methods. Mayo Clin Proc 65:584–596, 1990
57. Rickstein SE: Thoracic epidural analgesia and myocardial ischemia in the nonsurgical patient. Acta Anesths Scand 96s:87–89, 1991
58. Semsroth M, Hiesmayr M: Postoperative continuous application of morphine is more effective than bolus application for analgosedation in children. Anaesthesist 39:552–556, 1990
59. Tyler DC: Respiratory effects of pain in a child after thoracotomy. Anesthesiology 70:873–874, 1989

60. Benjamin JJ, Cascade PN, Rubenfire M, Wajszczuk W, Kerin NZ: Left lower lobe atelectasis and consolidation following cardiac surgery: The effect of topical cooling on the phrenic nerve. Radiology 142:11–14, 1982

61. Rosen K, Rosen D, Bank E: Caudal morphine for postop pain control in children undergoing cardiac procedures. Anesthesiology 67(3):a510, 1987

62. Pansard JL, Mankikian B, Clergue F: Thoracic epidural anesthesia and respiratory changes in diaphragmatic function after surgery. Acta Anesthesiol Scand 96s:90–93, 1991

63. Parfey NA, Moore W, Hutchins DMJ: Is pain crisis a cause of death in sickle cell disease. Clin Pathol 84:209–212, 1984

64. Anand KJS, Phil D, Carr DB, Hickey PR: Randomized trial of high dose sufentanil anesthesia in neonates undergoing cardiac surgery: Hormonal and hemodynamic stress response. Anesthesiology 67(3A): A501, 1987

65. Anand KJS, Phil D, Hickey PR: Randomized trial of high dose sufentanil anesthesia in neonates undergoing cardiac surgery: Effects on the metabolic stress response. Anesthesiology 67(3A):A502, 1987

66. Anand JS, Kanwal JS, Ansely-Green A: Measuring the severity of surgical stress in newborn infants. J Pediatr Surg 23:297–305, 1988

67. Anand KJS, Hansen DD, Hickey PR: Hormonal-metabolic stress responses in neonates undergoing cardiac surgery. Anesthesiology 73(4):661–670, 1990

68. Anand KJS, Hickey PR: Halothane-morphine compared with high dose sufentanil for anesthesia and postoperative analgesia in neonatal cardiac surgery. N Engl J Med 326(1):1–9, 1992

69. Rosen DA, Rosen KR, Bove EL: Anesthesia for hypoplastic left heart syndrome: An anesthetic protocol to improve outcome (abstr). American Academy of Pediatrics, Section on Anesthesiology, Program for Scientific Sessions 12, 1988

70. Asaph JW, Keppel JF: Midline sternotomy for the treatment of primary pulmonary neoplasms. Am J Surg 147:589–592, 1984

71. Brenner JI, Ringel RE, Berman MA: Cardiologic perspectives of chest pain in childhood: A referral problem? To whom? Pediatr Clin North Am 31(6):1241–1258, 1984

72. Cheitlin MD, DeCastr CM, Carlos M, McAllister HA: Sudden death as a complication of anomalous left coronary artery origin from the anterior sinus of valsalva: A not so minor congenital abnormality. Circulation 50:780–787, 1974

73. Maron BJ, Roberts WC, McAllister HA, et al: Sudden death in young athletes. Circulation 62:218–229, 1980

74. Bissett GS, Schwartz DC, Meyer RA et al: Clinical spectrum and long-term follow-up of isolated mitral valve prolapse in 119 children. Circulation 2:423–429, 1980

75. Kavey RE, Soundheimer HM, Blackman MS: Detection of dysrhythmia in pediatric patients with mitral valve prolapse. Circulation 62(3):582–587, 1980

76. Betriv A, Wigle ED, Felderhof CH et al: Prolapse of the posterior leaflet

of the mitral valve associated with secundum atrial septal defect. Am J Cardiol 35:363–369, 1975

77. Grift AG, Bolgiano CS, Cunningham J: Sensations during chest tube removal. Heart Lung 20:131–136, 1991

78. Kashani JH, Lababidi Z, Jones RS: Depression in children and adolescents with cardiovascular symptomatology: The significance of chest pain. J Am Acad Child Adolesc Psychiatry 21:187–189, 1982

79. Wall PD: The prevention of postoperative pain. Pain 33:289–290, 1988

80. Grunau RVE, Craig KD: Pain expressions in neonates: Facial action and cry. Pain 28:395–410, 1987

81. McGrath PJ, Johnson G, Goodman JT et al: The Children's Hospital of Eastern Ontario Pain Scale (CHEOPS). A behavioral scale for rating postoperative pain in children. In Fields HL, Dubner R, Cervero F (eds): Advances in Pain Research and Therapy, pp. 395–402. New York, Raven Press, 1985

82. Bhatt-Mehta V, Rosen DA: Management of acute pain in children. Clin Pharm 10:667–685, 1991

83. Beyer J: The Oucher: A user's manual and technical report. Denver, CO, University of Colorado Health Sciences Center, 1988

84. Melzack R: The McGill pain questionnaire. Major properties and scoring methods. Pain 1(3):277–299, 1975

85. Tessler M, Savedra M, Ward J et al: Children's language of pain. In Dubner R, Gebhart G, Bond M (eds): Pain Research and Clinical Management. Vol 3, pp. 348–353. Amsterdam, Elsevier, 1988

86. Manne SL, Jacobsen PB, Redd WH: Assessment of acute pain: Do self-report, parent ratings and nurse ratings measure the same phenomenon? Pain 48(1):45–52, 1992

87. Burge S, Eichhorn M, DeStefano A, Foley T, Hoothay F, Quinn D: How painful are postop incisions? Amer J Nurs 86(11):1263–1265, 1986

88. Woolf CJ, Wall PD: A dissociation between the analgesic and antinociceptive effects of morphine. Neurosci Lett 64:238, 1986

89. McGuire L, Dizard S: Managing pain in the young patient. Nursing (Horsham) 12(8):52, 54–57, 1982

90. Lloyd-Thomas AR: Pain management in the paediatric patient. Br J Anaesth 64:85–104, 1990

91. Bush JP, Holmbeck GN, Cockrell JL: Patterns of p.r.n. analgesic drug administration in children following elective surgery. J Pediatr Psychol 14(3):433–448, 1989

92. Lynn AM, Opheim KE, Tyler DC: Morphine infusion after pediatric cardiac surgery. Crit Care Med 12:863–866, 1984

93. Moldenour CC, Hug CC: Continuous infusion of fentanyl for cardiac surgery. Anesth Analg 01:200, 1982.

94. Koren G, Goresky G, Crean P, Klein J, MacLeod SM: Unexpected alterations in fentanyl pharmacokinetics in children undergoing cardiac surgery: Age related or disease related? Dev Pharmacol Ther 9(3):183–191, 1986

95. Broadman LM, Rice LJ, Vaughan M, Ruttimann UE, Pollack MM: Parent assisted "PCA" for postoperative pain control in young children. Anesth Analg 70:S34, 1990

96. Ready LB: Patient controlled analgesia—Does it provide more than comfort? Can J Anaesth 37(7):719–721, 1990
97. Lange MP, Dahn MS, Jacobs LA: Patient-controlled analgesia versus intermittent analgesia dosing. Heart Lung 17:495–498, 1988
98. Aitken HA, Kenny GN: Use of patient-controlled analgesia in postoperative cardiac surgical patients. A survey of ward staff attitudes. Intensive Care Nurs 6(2):74–78, 1990
99. King KB, Norsen LH, Robertson RK, Hicks GL: Patient management of pain medication after cardiac surgery. Nurs Res 36(3):145–150, 1987
100. Berde CB, Yee JD, Lehn BM, Moore LJ, Sethan NF: Patient-controlled analgesia in children and adolescents: A randomized comparison with intramuscular morphine. Anesthesiology 73(3A):A1102, 1990
101. El-Baz N, Goldin M: Continuous epidural infusion of morphine for pain relief after cardiac operations. J Thorac Cardiovasc Surg 93:878–883, 1987
102. Shulman M, Sandler AN, Bradley JW, Young PS, Brebner J: Postthoracotomy pain and pulmonary function following epidural and systemic morphine. Anesthesiology 61:569–575, 1984
103. Asantila R, Rosenberg PH, Scheinin B: Comparison of different methods of postoperative analgesia after thoracotomy. Acta Anesthesiol Scand 30:421–425, 1986
104. Rosen KR, Rosen DA: Caudal epidural morphine for control of pain following open-heart surgery in children. Anesthesiology 70:418–421, 1989
105. Fitzpatrick GJ, Moriarty DC: Intrathecal morphine in the management of pain following cardiac surgery: A comparison with morphine i.v. Br J Anaesth 60(6):639–644, 1988
106. Bosenberg AT, Bland BA, Schulte-Steinberg O, Downing JW: Thoracic epidural anesthesia via caudal route in infants. Anesthesiology 69(2):265–269, 1988
107. Gray JR, Fromme GA, Nauss LA, Wang JK, Ilstrup DM: Intrathecal morphine for post-thoracotomy pain. Anesth Analg 65:873–876, 1986
108. Krane EJ, Tyler DC, Jacobson LE: The dose response of caudal morphine in children. Anesthesiology 71:48–52, 1989
109. Fischer RL, Lubenow TR, Liceaga A, McCarthy RJ, Ivankovich AD: Comparison of continuous epidural infusion of fentanyl-bupivacaine and morphine-bupivacaine in management of postoperative pain. Anesth Analg 67:559–563, 1988
110. Takasaki M, Dohi S, Kawabata Y, Takahashi T: Dosage of lidocaine for caudal anesthesia in infants and children. Anesthesiology 47:527–529, 1977
111. Desparmet J, Meistelman C, Barre J, Saint-Maurice C: Continuous epidural infusion of bupivacaine for postoperative pain relief in children. Anesthesiology 67:108–110, 1987
112. Chien BB, Burke RG, Hunter DJ: An extensive experience with postoperative pain relief using postoperative fentanyl infusion. Arch Surg 126:692–694, 1991
113. Glass PS, Estok P, Ginsberg B, Goldberg JS, Sladen RN: Use of patient-controlled analgesia to compare the efficacy of epidural to intravenous fentanyl administration. Anesth Analg 74:345–351, 1992

114. Robinson RJ, Brister S, Jones E, Quigly M: Epidural meperidine analgesia after cardiac surgery. Can Anaesth Soc J 33:550–555, 1986

115. Patrick JA, Meyer-Witting M, Reynold F: Lumbar epidural diamorphine following thoracic surgery. A comparison of infusion and bolus administration. Anaesthesia 46(2):85–89, 1991

116. Magora F, Chrubasik J, Damm D, Schulte-Monting J, Shir Y: Application of a new method for measurement of plasma methadone levels to the use of epidural methadone for relief of postoperative pain. Anesth Analg 66:1308–1311, 1987

117. Jones SEF, Beasley JM, McFarlane DWR, Davis JM, Hall-Davies G: Intrathecal morphine for postoperative pain relief in children. Br J Anaesth 56:137–140, 1984

118. Krane EJ: Delayed respiratory depression in a child after caudal epidural morphine. Anesth Analg 67:79–82, 1988

119. McIlvaine W: Spinal opioids for the pediatric patient. J Pain Symptom Manage 5(3):183–190, 1990

120. Naji P, Farschtschian M, Wilder-Smith OH, Wilder-Smith CH: Epidural droperidol and morphine for postoperative pain. Anesth Analg 70:583–588, 1990

121. Lawhorn CD, Galladay S, Brown RE, Andelman P: Epidural morphine with butorphenol for postoperative analgesia in pediatric patients undergoing thoracic procedures. Anesth Analg 74:S177, 1992

122. Vanstrum GS, Bjornson KM, Ilko R: Postoperative effects of intrathecal morphine in coronary artery bypass surgery. Anesth Analg 67:261–267, 1988

123. Rosen KR, Rosen DA, Callow L, Bove EL, Reynolds PI, Shayevitz JR, Malviya SV, Wilton NCT, Lupinetti FM, Bhatt-Mehta V, Meliones JN: Caudal epidural morphine for control of postoperative pain in children undergoing cardiac surgery (abstr). Submitted to the Section on Anesthesiology, American Academy of Pediatrics, 1992

124. Koren G, Goresky G, Crean P, Klein J, Macleod SM: Pediatric fentanyl dosing based on pharmacokinetics during cardiac surgery. Anesth Analg 63:577–582, 1984

125. Rosen D, Rosen K, Davidson B, Broadman L: Fentanyl uptake by the Scimed membrane oxygenator. J Cardiothoracic Vasc Anesth 2:619–620, 1988

126. Bellamy CD, McDonnell FJ, Colclough GW, Walmsley PN, Hine JM, Jarecky TW, Vanderveer BL: Epidural infusion/PCA for pain control in pediatric patients. Anesth Analg 70:S19, 1990

127. Marlow S, Engstrom R, White PF: Epidural patient-controlled analgesia (PCA). An alternative to continuous epidural infusions. Pain 37:97–101, 1989

128. Miguel R, Trimble G: Patient-controlled epidural analgesia: Efficient and effective postoperative analgesia! Anesthesiology 73(3A):A795, 1990

129. Grant RP, Dolman JF, Harper JA, White SA, Parsons DG, Evans KG, Merrick P: Patient-controlled lumbar epidural fentanyl for post thoracotomy pain. Can J Anaesth 37:s45, 1990

130. Ellis R, Haines D, Shah R, Cotton BR, Smith G: Pain relief after abdominal surgery—A comparison of intramuscular morphine, sublingual

buprenorphine and self-administered intravenous pethidine. Br J Anaesth 54:421–428, 1982

131. Hånning CD, Vickers AP, Smith G, Graham NB, McNiel ME: The morphine hydrogel suppository. A new sustained release rectal preparation. Br J Anaesth 61:221–228, 1988

132. Rowbotham DJ, Wyld R, Peacock JE, Duthie DJR, Nimmo WJ: Transdermal fentanyl for the relief of pain after upper abdominal surgery. Br J Anaesth 63:56–59, 1989

133. Mannuksela EL, Kokki H: Efficacy of intravenous keterolac compared with morphine in relieving postoperative pain in children (abstr). Section on Anesthesiology, American Academy of Pediatrics: p. 41, 1992

134. Watcha MF, Jones MB, Lagueruela RG, Schweiger C, White PF: Comparison of keterolac and morphine as adjuvants during pediatric surgery. Anesthesiology 76(3):368–372, 1992

135. Woodring JH, Royer JM, Todd EP: Upper rib fractures following median sternotomy. Ann Thorac Surg 39(4):355–357, 1985

136. Restelli L, Movilia P, Bossi L, Caironi C: Management of pain after thoracotomy: A technique of multiple intercostal nerve blocks. Anesthesiology 61:353–354, 1984

137. de la Rocha AG, Chambers K: Pain amelioration after thoracotomy: A prospective randomized study. Ann Thorac Surg 37(3):239–242, 1984

138. Baker JW, Tribble CG: Pleural anesthetics given through an epidural catheter secured inside a chest tube. Ann Thorac Surg 51(1):138–139, 1991

139. Eisenach JC, Lysak SZ, Viscomi CM: Epidural clonidine analgesia following surgery: Phase 1. Anesthesiology 71:640–646, 1989

140. Gordh T: A study on the analgesic effect of clonidine in man. Acta Anaesthesiol Scand 27:72, 1983

141. von Bormann B, Boldt J, Strum G, Kling D, Weidler B, Lohmann E, Hempelmann G: Calcium-antagonists in anaesthesia. Additive analgesia caused by nimodipin in cardiosurgical interventions. Anaesthesist 34:429–434, 1985

142. Bafford DC: Progressive relaxation as a nursing intervention: A method of controlling pain for open-heart surgery patients. Commun Nurs Res 8:284–290, 1977

143. McCaffery M: Pain relief for the child. Pediatr Nurs 3:11–16, 1977

144. Carlsson CA, Persson K, Pelletieri L: Painful scars after thoracic and abdominal surgery. Acta Chir Scand 151:309–311, 1985

145. Navarathnam RG, Wang IYS, Thomas D, Klineberg PL: Evaluation of the transcutaneous electrical nerve stimulator for postoperative analgesia following cardiac surgery. Anaesth Intensive Care 12:345–350, 1984

146. Mindus P: Anxiety, pain and sedation. Acta Anaesthesiol Scand 32(S88):7–12, 1987

147. Egbert LD, Battit GE, Welch CE, Marshall KB: Reduction in postoperative pain by encouragement and instruction of patients. N Engl J Med 270(16):825–827, 1964

148. Lane JC, Tennison MB, Lawless ST, Greenwood RS, Zaritsky AL: Movement disorders after withdrawal of fentanyl infusion. J Pediatr 119(4):664–671, 1991

149. Bergman I, Steeves M, Burckart G, Thompson A: Reversible neurologic abnormalities associated with prolonged intravenous midazolam and fentanyl administration. J Pediatr 119:644–649, 1991

150. Shafer A, White PF, Schuttler J, Rosenthal MH: Use of fentanyl infusion in the intensive care unit: Tolerance to its anaesthetic effects. Anesthesiology 59:245–248, 1983

151. Arnold JH, Truog RD, Scavone JM, Fenton T: Changes in pharmacodynamic response to fentanyl in neonates during continuous infusion. J Pediatr 119(4):639–643, 1991

152. Joaschimsson PO, Hedstrand U, Eklund A: Low dose ketamine infusion for analgesia during postoperative ventilator treatment. Acta Anaesthesiol Scand 30:697–702, 1986

153. Owen H, Reekie RM, Clements JA, Watson R, Nimmo WS: Analgesia from morphine and ketamine. Anaesthesia 42:1051–1056, 1987

154. Tobias JD, Martin LD, Wetzel RC: Ketamine by continuous infusion for sedation in the pediatric intensive care unit. Crit Care Med 18(8):819–821, 1990

155. Rosen DA, Rosen KR, Custer J, Koopmann C, Meliones J: Midazolam and ketamine: A special sedative when spontaneous ventilation is needed (abstr). Pediatric Critical Care Colloquium, October 3, 1990

156. Rosen DA, Rosen KR: Pain and sedation in the pediatric patient: The 1990 approach to a very old problem. In Vincent JL (ed): Update in Intensive Care and Emergency Medicine. Update 1990, pp. 758–769. Berlin, Germany, Springer-Verlag, 1990

157. Aitekenhead AR: Analgesia and sedation in intensive care. Br J Anaesth 63(2):196–206, 1989

158. Grounds RM, Lalor JM, Lumley J, Royston D, Morgan M: Propofol infusion for sedation in the intensive care: A preliminary report. BMJ 294:397–400, 1987

159. McMurray TJ, Collier PS, Carson IW, Lyons SM, Elliot P: Propofol sedation after open heart surgery: A clinical and pharmakokinetic study. Anaesthesia 45:322–326, 1990

160. Baeuerle JJ, Kinsley CP, Ward JA, Williams D, Hinds J: The effect of propofol on myocardial contractility and function in normovolemic and hypovolemic swine. Anesth Analg 74(25):S14, 1992

161. Au J, Walker WS, Scott DHT: Withdrawal syndrome after propofol infusion. Anaesthesia 45:741–742, 1990

162. Wildsmith JAW: Aspects of pain. Br J Anaesth 63(2):135, 1989

Pain Management in Cardiothoracic Surgery, edited by Gravlee and Rauck. J. B. Lippincott Company, Philadelphia © 1993.

Kevin L. Speight

6 | Perioperative Stress Response Suppression in Cardiothoracic Surgery

Postoperative stress is the term generally used to describe the continuation of the normal stress response to surgical injury into the postoperative period. Stress response (or general adaptive response) refers to the biochemical and physiologic adaptation made by an organism, presumably to allow for improved survival after injury.

Overall, in the physician community in general and the anesthesiologist community in particular, there is a bias that the same response tailored to increase survival "in the wild" may be harmful to the surgically injured patient. Interest by the medical community in this dilemma is evidenced by the amount of material published about it in the last decade and the proliferation of anesthetic techniques touted to reduce "stress." Pain services to manage postoperative pain partly represent an outgrowth of the belief that stress reduction in the postoperative period is critical.

The bias that modification of stress response may benefit surgical patients rests on widely held premises that often go unstated: (1) stress response was adaptive for injury "in the wild," (2) stress response in managed injury (surgery) can be destructive, (3) stress response begins with surgery and continues into the postoperative period, (4) stress response can be modified by various "anesthetic manipulations, (5) stress response can be quantitated by various biochemical and physiologic measurements, and (6) reduction of "measured stress response" should be related to improved outcome.

THE STRESS RESPONSE

The teleological significance of the stress response for human beings probably lies in the evolution of humans as a "hunter-gatherer."[1] On receiving an injury that limits mobility, survival depends on rapid restoration of the ability to ambulate. The stress response in humans consists of: (1) mobilization of stored energy sources, (2) provision of a biochemical milieu for rapid repair of the injured structure, and (3) retention of substances essential for life (water and energy), all of

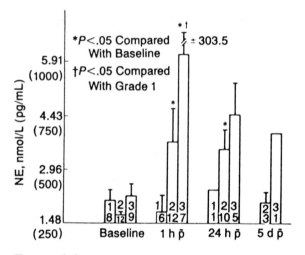

FIGURE 6–1.   Stress hormone levels before surgery and at 1 hour, 24 hours, and 5 days after surgery. The bars for each time period represent (in order) minor, moderate, and severe surgical procedures (stress). Higher intensities of surgical stress elicit norepinephrine levels that are higher than baseline values at 1 hour and at 24 hours. (A) Norepinephrine (NE) levels are different between the moderate and severe stress groups at 1 hour. Numbers 1, 2, and 3 in bars indicate groups (1 = mild, 2 = moderate, and 3 = severe). The second (lower) number in each bar indicates the number of patients in group. (B) Moderate and severe surgical stresses cause significant elevations of epinephrine levels at 1 hour which return to baseline by 24 hours. (C) Moderate and severe stresses cause significant elevations of cortisol from baseline at 1 hour. Severe stress causes cortisol levels that are different from baseline at 24 hours postoperatively. (*Reprinted with permission from Chernow et al. Arch Intern Med 147:1273–1278, 1987*)

which subserve rapid return to ambulation. When a person is injured a cascade of events occurs yielding the "ebb and flow" of the stress response as described by Cuthbertson.[1] Injury information is transmitted to peripheral nerves via mechanoreceptor and nociceptive receptors in the tissue. Local factors such as prostanoids and kinins augment this response and begin the inflammatory process at the local level. Through adrenergic transmission, the peripheral nerve conducts information regarding tissue injury to the spinal cord. Reflexly, at the spinal cord level, activation of the sympathetic nervous system occurs and injury information is transmitted to the brain. The brain responds by release of trophic factors for endocrine response and neural impulses that complete the stress response.

The time course of the stress response has been reported in a number of studies.[2-6] Figures 6–1, 6–2, and 6–3 show norepinephrine, epinephrine, and cortisol levels with various grades of surgical stimulation over 5 days. Plasma epinephrine, norepinephrine, and cortisol levels increase within 1 hour of all but the most superficial surgeries. Epinephrine levels return to baseline within 24 hours while norepinephrine and cortisol tend to remain elevated at 24 hours and

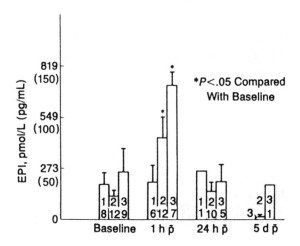

FIGURE 6–2.   Epinephrine levels before surgery and at 1 hour, 24 hours, and 5 days after surgery. The bars for each time period represent (in order) minor, moderate, and severe surgical procedures (stress). Moderate and severe surgical stresses cause significant elevations of epinephrine levels at 1 hour which return to baseline by 24 hours. (*Reprinted with permission from Chernow et al. Arch Intern Med 147:1273–1278, 1987*)

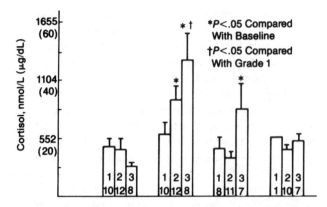

FIGURE 6–3.　Cortisol levels before surgery and at 1 hour, 24 hours, and 5 days after surgery. The bars for each time period represent (in order) minor, moderate, and severe surgical procedures (stress). Moderate and severe stresses cause significant elevations of cortisol from baseline at 1 hour. Severe stress causes cortisol levels that are different from baseline at 24 hours post operatively. *(Reprinted with permission from Chernow et al. Arch Intern Med 147:1273–1278, 1987)*

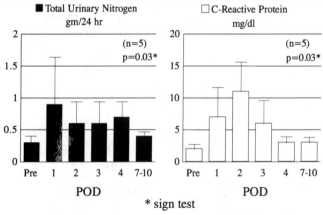

FIGURE 6–4.　Total urinary nitrogen and plasma C-reactive protein levels in neonates after surgery show trends toward increases at postoperative days 1 through 3. *(Reprinted with permission from Chwals, Dept. of General Surgery, The Bowman Gray School of Medicine of Wake Forest University)*

TABLE 6–1. Urinary Excretion of Epinephrine and Norepinephrine After Gastrectomy

	Preoperative Day	Day of Operation	Postoperative Day 1	Postoperative Day 2	Postoperative Day 3
Epinephrine					
General (n = 17)	4.1 ± 0.6[a]	35.4 ± 7.2	14.9 ± 2.2	9.2 ± 1.7	5.4 ± 2.4[b]
Epidural (n = 17)	4.4 ± 0.8	11.1 ± 1.9	13.3 ± 1.7	10.3 ± 1.4	7.7 ± 2.3
P	N.S.	<0.01	N.S.	N.S.	N.S.
Norepinephrine					
General (n = 17)	30.0 ± 3.2	71.4 ± 9.7	109.6 ± 10.9	112.4 ± 15.2	65.6 ± 14.7[b]
Epidural (n = 17)	40.5 ± 6.8	42.6 ± 5.6	66.8 ± 6.9	68.5 ± 8.0	54.5 ± 4.0[b]
P	N.S.	<0.05	<0.01	<0.05	N.S.

[a]values (mcg/day) are expressed as mean ± SEM.
[b]n = 8
P significance level of difference between the two group
N.S. not significant
(Reprinted with permission from Tsuji et al. Jpn J Surg 12:344–348, 1982)

return to baseline within 5 days. The metabolic response of infants to surgical stress (reported by Chwals) reflects this time course and is represented in Figure 6–4.[5] Table 6–1 shows the time course of epinephrine response to surgical stimulus as reported by Tsuji and Shiraska.[2]

Seitz recently compared the stress hormone response during anesthesia and surgery using a variety of general anesthetic techniques (Figs. 6–5, 6–6, 6–7, 6–8).[4] These data support a rapid rise in plasma catecholamine and cortisol levels despite general anesthesia.

One must also graft an understanding of the organism's initial functional state to the knowledge of the usual neuroendocrine response to surgical injury. The state of the organism before injury can

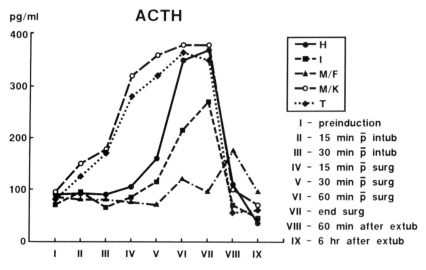

FIGURE 6–5.   Adrenocorticotropic hormone levels with various general anesthetic techniques at various times preoperation, during surgery, and after completion of surgery. (I = preinduction, II = 15 minutes after intubation, III = 30 minutes after intubation, IV = 15 minutes after incision, V = 30 minutes after incision, VI = 60 minutes after incision, VII = end of surgery, VIII = 60 minutes after extubation, IX = 6 hours after extubation) Agents are indicated by letter abbreviation and all include use of nitrous oxide/oxygen (H = halothane, I = isoflurane, M/F = midazolam/fentanyl, M/K = midazolam/ketamine, T = tramadol). (*Reprinted with permission from Seitz et al. Anaesthesiol Reanim 16:147–158, 1991*)

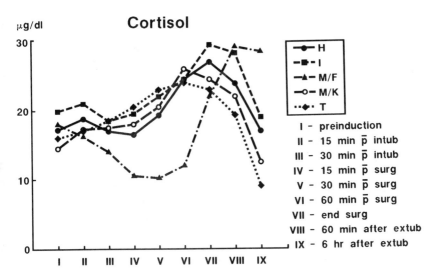

FIGURE 6–6. Cortisol levels with various general anesthetic techniques at various times preoperation, during surgery, and after completion of surgery. (I = preinduction, II = 15 minutes after intubation, III = 30 minutes after intubation, IV = 15 minutes after incision, V = 30 minutes after incision, VI = 60 minutes after incision, VII = end of surgery, VIII = 60 minutes after extubation, IX = 6 hours after extubation) Agents are indicated by letter abbreviation and all include use of nitrous oxide/oxygen (H = halothane, I = isoflurane, M/F = midazolam/fentanyl, M/K = midazolam/ketamine, T = tramadol). (*Reprinted with permission from Seitz et al. Anaesthesiol Reanim 16:147–158, 1991*)

modify the form of the stress response or change the ability to respond. Examples of such preexisting conditions include cardiac or pulmonary dysfunction, whether the preexisting end-organ compromise is congenital or acquired. Figure 6–9 illustrates the impact of initial functional state in the rapidly growing preterm neonate. A preterm infant between 28 to 32 weeks postconceptual age responds to injury stress with near total arrest of growth as measured by body weight, crown-rump length, and head circumference changes. Because of the growth stoppage, caloric requirements of a sick infant may actually fall below those of a healthy neonate.[5] This is in contradistinction to adults, in whom any significant stress increases metabolic rate and caloric requirements. Figure 6–10 illustrates the pitfall that meets the aged or physiologically compromised patient subjected

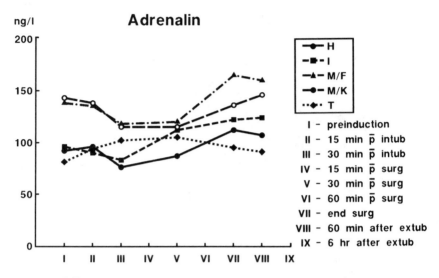

FIGURE 6–7. Epinephrine levels with various general anesthetic techniques at various times preoperation, during surgery, and after completion of surgery. (I = preinduction, II = 15 minutes after intubation, III = 30 minutes after intubation, IV = 15 minutes after incision, V = 30 minutes after incision, VI = 60 minutes after incision, VII = end of surgery, VIII = 60 minutes after extubation, IX = 6 hours after extubation) Agents are indicated by letter abbreviation and all include use of nitrous oxide/oxygen (H = halothane, I = isoflurane, M/F = midazolam/fentanyl, M/K = midazolam/ketamine, T = tramadol). *(Reprinted with permission from Seitz et al. Anaesthesiol Reanim 16:147–158, 1991)*

to stress.[3] During the period of stress response in experimental stress models, humans demonstrate 20% to 30% increases in cardiac output, oxygen consumption, carbon dioxide elimination, and metabolic rate. In an organism with limited physiological reserve, these stresses may cause organ failure resulting in morbidity or mortality.

In summary, the stress response serves to preserve scarce resources (energy and water) and remobilize the injured organism. The time course of the stress response relates to the period of ongoing injury as long as the organism is able to respond. The stress response is characterized by both biochemical (catecholamine, cortisol, etc.) and physiologic changes (increased oxygen uptake, carbon dioxide elimination, cardiac output, and metabolic rate), based on the organism's starting condition. The response to stress can be predicted to

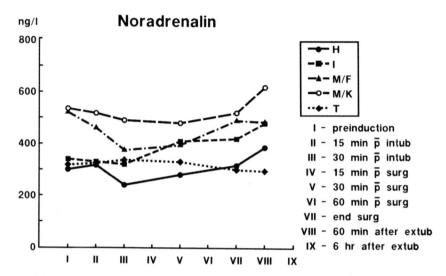

FIGURE 6–8.   Norepinephrine levels with various general anesthetic techniques at various times preoperation, during surgery, and after completion of surgery. (I = preinduction, II = 15 minutes after intubation, III = 30 minutes after intubation, IV = 15 minutes after incision, V = 30 minutes after incision, VI = 60 minutes after incision, VII = end of surgery, VIII = 60 minutes after extubation, IX = 6 hours after extubation) Agents are indicated by letter abbreviation and all include use of nitrous oxide/oxygen (H = halothane, I = isoflurane, M/F = midazolam/fentanyl, M/K = midazolam/ketamine, T = tramadol). *(Reprinted with permission from Seitz et al. Anaesthesiol Reanim 16:147–158, 1991)*

some degree. Limited physiologic reserve before injury or special circumstances such as rapid growth may significantly alter the organism's response to stress. An unbridled stress response may cause morbidity or death in an organism unable to meet the required physiologic demands.

MODIFICATION OF THE STRESS RESPONSE

General anesthesia had its roots in the public demonstration of ether in the United States in the 1840s. Concurrent to the use of ether in the United States, the use of chloroform as a general anesthetic was described in Britain. Nearly a century later, in the early 1900s, Cuth-

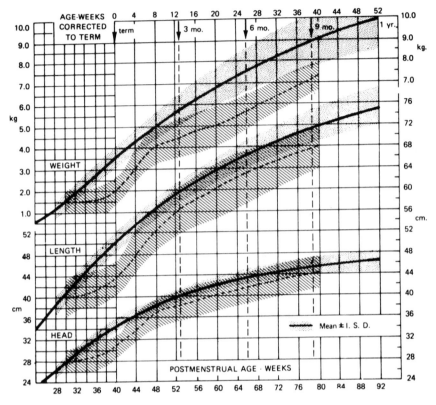

FIGURE 6–9. Growth is arrested during the stress of illness in the 28th to 32nd postconceptual week. Diagonal shading represents growth of sick preterm infants, and solid lines represent Babson's curves for postnatal growth in well infants. Between the 28th and 32nd postconceptual week illness is attended by nearly complete arrest in dimensional and weight growth. *(Reprinted with permission from Maisels et al. J Pediatr 98:663, 1981)*

bertson began the work that underlies our current understanding of the biochemical changes occurring during the metabolic response to stress.[1]

Increases in traumatic disease attendant with world wars and industrialized society, combined with the common acceptance of surgery for many pathologic disorders, has placed pressure on medicine to develop knowledge interrelating anesthesia and the metabolic response to trauma. Knowledge of this field continues to grow.

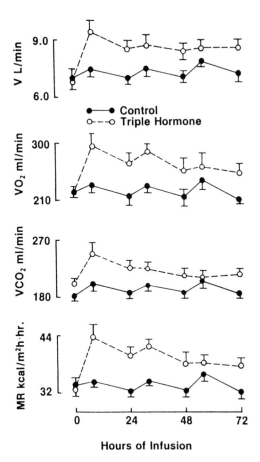

Hours of Infusion

FIGURE 6–10. "Triple hormone" infusion (cortisol, glucagon, and epinephrine) in volunteers showing effects on physiologic parameters versus control (saline infusion) group. Ventilation, oxygen consumption, carbon dioxide production, and metabolic rate all increase significantly in the hormone infusion group (amount of increase approximately 30 + %). *(Reprinted with permission from Bessey et al. Ann Surg 200:264–281, 1984)*

TABLE 6–2.   Anesthetic Dose, Patient Norepinephrine Responses, and Calculated Doses Blocking Adrenergic Response

	MAC Multiple/Morphine Dose (mg/kg)[a]				MAC BAR$_{50}$[b]	MAC BAR$_{95}$
	1.0	1.3/0.4	1.6/0.9	1.9/1.4		
Enflurane	—	34 (9)[c]	43 (14)	73 (11)	1.60 ± 0.13 MAC	2.57 MAC
Halothane	0 (6)	42 (12)	56 (9)	87 (15)	1.45 ± 0.08 MAC	2.10 MAC
Morphine	—	0 (8)	13 (8)	87 (8)	1.13 ± 0.09 mg/kg plus 60% N$_2$O	1.45 mg/kg plus 60% N$_2$O

a,b,cIn the cell under MAC multiple/morphine dose are the percentages of patients who did not have a significant plasma norepinephrine level change from baseline with surgical manipulation. In parenthesis are the number of patients studied in each group. MAC BARs are the calculated doses of anesthetics (administered with 60% nitrous oxide) that would prevent significant norepinephrine responses in 50% of the population. (Reprinted with permission from Roizen et al. Anesthesiology 54:390–399, 1981)

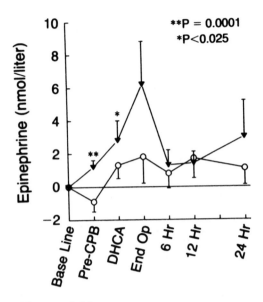

FIGURE 6–11. Changes in plasma epinephrine levels from baseline with either halothane (triangles) or sufentanil (open circles) during different stages of surgery and after surgery for congenital heart lesion repair. *(Reproduced with permission from Anand et al. N Engl J Med 326:1–9, 1992)*

GENERAL ANESTHESIA AND THE STRESS RESPONSE

General anesthetic drugs have developed along three main themes: volatile anesthetics (halocarbons and substituted ethers), narcotics (of different potencies and pharmacokinetics), and a group of substances loosely classified as sedative–hypnotics (barbiturates, benzodiazepines, etc). Adjuvants have been added to these differing anesthetic drugs, most notably muscle relaxants. Today's "balanced general anesthetic" is commonly produced with a combination of a number of different drugs administered to render a patient immobile, amnestic, analgesic, and hemodynamically stable during the period of operation. That there are differences in these concoctions of "general anesthetics" with respect to intraoperative stress response is not surprising.

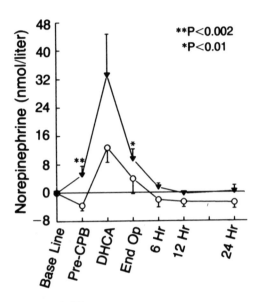

FIGURE 6–12.   Changes in plasma norepinephrine levels from baseline with either halothane (triangles) or sufentanil (open circles)
during different stages of surgery and after surgery for congenital heart lesion repair. *(Reproduced with permission from Anand et al. N Engl
J Med 326:1–9, 1992)*

In 1981 Roizen et al. presented information relating anesthetic
dose to the ability to block autonomic responses.[7] Table 6–2 shows
data comparing three techniques of general anesthesia and the doses
required to block plasma catecholamine increases to surgical stimulation. Roizen and his colleagues concluded that the endocrine response to stimulus is a function of the depth of anesthesia, and that
reporting the endocrine stress response without regard to the potency of anesthetic (MAC) is illogical. Roizen's pioneering work
showed the dose ranges at which several general anesthetics block
autonomic responses. Anand and colleagues[8–10] have added to Roizen's
work by comparing different "usual and customary" anesthetics in a
particular population (pediatrics undergoing heart surgery). These
studies showed significantly different endocrine stress responses
(Figs. 6–11, 6–12, and 6–13) with commonly used anesthetic regimens. Anand and Hickey feel that there are significant differences in

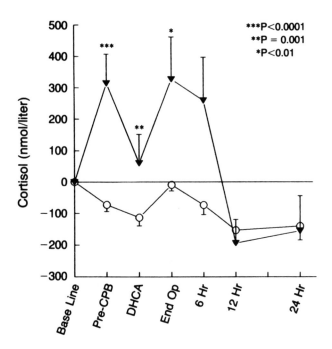

FIGURE 6–13.   Changes in plasma cortisol levels from
baseline with either halothane (triangles) or sufentanil (open
circles) during different stages of surgery and after surgery for
congenital heart lesion repair. *(Reproduced with permission
from Anand et al. N Engl J Med 326:1–9, 1992)*

both morbid and mortal events (Table 6–3) that can be related to reduction of stress response in their study population.[9] Crozier et al.
reported similar hormonal responses in an adult population (Tables
6–4 and 6–5) comparing commonly used general anesthetic techniques.[11] Crozier et al. did not relate measured stress response differences to outcome in their study population as did Anand and Hickey.
Seitz recently compared the hormonal patterns among commonly
used general anesthetics (halothane/nitrous oxide, isoflurane/nitrous
oxide, midazolam/fentanyl/nitrous oxide, midazolam/ketamine/nitrous
oxide, and tramadol/nitrous oxide) during surgery[4] and concluded
that different anesthetic techniques could provide adequate surgical
conditions while differing significantly in the degree of stress response blockade.

TABLE 6–3.   Postoperative Complications and Outcome in the Two Groups of Neonates [a]

Finding	Halothane Group (N = 15)	Sufentanil Group (N = 30)	P Value[b]
Hypotension	11 (73)	13 (43)	0.055
Arrhythmias	7 (47)	6 (20)	0.154
Sepsis or necrotizing enterocolitis	3 (20)	0	0.032
Disseminated intravascular coagulation	3 (20)	0	0.032
Seizures	4 (27)	3 (10)	0.154
Metabolic acidosis	4 (27)	0	0.009
Death	4 (27)	0	0.009
Postoperative ventilation (hr)	125 ± 45[c]	127 ± 21	0.086[d]
Postoperative ICU stay (days)	9.0 ± 2.0[c]	8.6 ± 0.9	0.413[d]
Postoperative hospital stay (days)	16.1 ± 3.6[c]	16.9 ± 2.3	0.214[d]

[a]Plus–minus values are means ± SE. Values in parentheses are percentages.
[b]By Fisher's exact test except as noted.
[c]Data on the 11 surviving infants are given.
[d]By the Mann–Whitney U test.
(Reproduced with permission from Anand et al. N. Engl J Med 326:1–9, 1992)

SUBARACHNOID AND EPIDURAL BLOCKADE AND STRESS RESPONSE

Initially there was much debate about the ability to block stress hormones during surgery with epidural or subarachnoid (spinal) anesthesia.[12–19] The present consensus is that epidural or spinal blocks of sufficient density and height reduce stress markers as compared with general anesthetics using volatile agents or sedative hypnotics. However, there is some indication that spinal or epidural blocks may be no more effective in reducing the stress response than moderate doses of potent opioids (Figs. 6–14, 6–15, 6–16, and Table 6–6).[20] Local anesthetics are required in the epidural or subarachnoid space for maximal suppression of stress responses, as compared with epidural or subarachnoid narcotics alone.[15–18,19,21,22]

Epidural opioids appear to have a distinct advantage over intravenous opioids if reduction of stress response is desirable in the post-

TABLE 6–4. Changes in Plasma Catecholamine Levels (median and range)

Point	Halothane Group (pmol/l)	Fentanyl Group (pmol/l)	Difference Between Groups (Mann–Whitney U test)
1 E	123 (77–268)	93 (20–320)	n.s.
NE	175 (101–364)	172 (20–236)	n.s.
2 E	43 (20–72)[a]	39 (20–75)[c]	n.s.
NE	215 (121–452)[a]	102 (55–152)[a]	n.s.
3 E	48 (20–94)[a]	42 (20–192)[c]	n.s.
NE	163 (90–290)[a]	95 (62–182)[b]	P < 0.01
4 E	136 (60–720)[c]	194 (32–342)[b,g]	n.s.
NE	457 (232–795)[d]	293 (109–558)[d]	P < 0.05
5 E	222 (61–626)[c]	94 (33–411)[a,g]	P < 0.01
NE	425 (235–598)[d]	190 (113–649)[b]	n.s.
6 E	298 (75–778)[c]	218 (80–1042)[b,e]	n.s.
NE	425 (144–878)[c]	307 (162–457)[b]	P < 0.05
7 E	469 (83–1587)[c]	760 (187–2840)[d,g]	n.s.
NE	477 (233–1504)[c]	662 (305–1537)[d]	n.s.
8 E	325 (95–611)[c]	388 (120–1112)[d,g]	n.s.
NE	390 (320–542)[c]	360 (193–934)[c]	n.s.

Symbols:
E = epinephrine, NE = norepinephrine
[a]P < 0.1; [b]P < 0.05; [c]P < 0.01; [d]P < 0.001 compared to point 1. [e]P < 0.05, [f]P < 0.01, [g]P < 0.001 compared to point 3.
n.s. = not significant
(Point 1 = preinduction, 2 & 3 = 5 and 30 minutes postinduction without surgical stimulation, 4 = with peritoneal retractors in place and before gut manipulation, 5 = maximal gut stimulation, 6 = during wound closure, 7 & 8 = 30 and 120 minutes after the end of surgery). (Reproduced with permission from Crozier et al. Horm Metab Res 20:352–356, 1988)

operative period. Epidural analgesia can be continued into the post-operative period, giving pain relief with less sedation than would be present with the levels of intravenous potent opioids that would be required to block the stress response.

AUTONOMIC AND PERIPHERAL BLOCKADE AND THE STRESS RESPONSE

Scientific information relating peripheral autonomic blockade or peripheral somatic blockade to the stress response is more limited than that available for general, epidural, or spinal anesthetics. Chari reported some diminution in cortisol levels (during the period of local anesthetic action) if celiac plexus blocks were performed prior to ab-

TABLE 6–5. Changes in Cortisol Plasma Levels (mean and SD)

Point	Halothane Group (pmol/l)	Fentanyl Group (pmol/l)	Differences Between Groups (Mann–Whitney U test)
1	6.2 (3.6–11.4)	4.4 (1.5–5.7)	n.s.
2	6.8 (1.9–9.9)[a]	3.0 (0.8–6.9)[a]	$P < 0.05$
3	6.6 (1.7–17.7)[a]	1.9 (0.2–4.5)[c]	$P < 0.05$
4	29.0 (16.3–48.7)[c]	5.7 (1.6–17.6)[a]	$P < 0.001$
5	36.6 (17.4–65.4)[c]	15.2 (2.1–25.8)[c]	$P < 0.001$
6	33.9 (20.3–63.6)[b]	16.2 (13.0–25.2)[b]	$P < 0.01$
7	42.7 (19.6–51.1)[c]	18.9 (14.2–28.2)[c]	$P < 0.01$
8	41.9 (29.4–66.0)[c]	24.0 (12.1–34.3)[c]	$P < 0.05$

Symbols:
Student's t-test for paired samples, each point is compared to point 1:
[a] $P > 0.1$; [b] $P < 0.05$; [c] $P < 0.01$
n.s. = not significant
(Reproduced with permission from Crozier et al. Horm Metab Res 20:352–356, 1988)

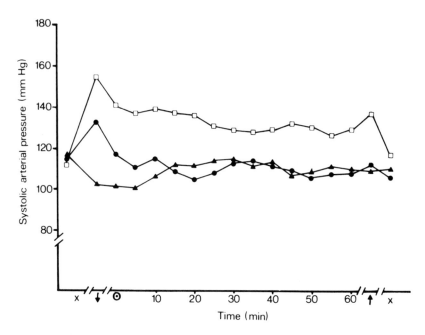

FIGURE 6–14. Systolic arterial pressure during the course of induction, surgery, and emergence with intravenous althesin alone (open squares), althesin with spinal anesthesia (blackened circles) or althesin with fentanyl (blackened triangles). On the x-axis, xs mark the beginning and end of anesthesia, the downward arrow indicates tracheal intubation, the circle enclosing a dot indicates skin incision, and tracheal extubation is indicated by the upward arrow. *(Reproduced with permission from Blunnie et al. Br J Anaesth 55:611–618, 1983)*

dominal surgery.[23] Interpleural blocks, which are (in effect) intercostal nerve blocks, have not been shown to alter stress response to abdominal surgery.[24] Little information exists about stress response and extremity blocks (e.g., brachial plexus block) but it would seem logical that blocking an extremity would prevent neural traffic normally responsible for the stress response. The reality that peripheral surgeries are usually not as stimulating as procedures on body cavities complicates the comparison between regional anesthesia and general anesthesia regarding modification of the stress response to peripheral surgery. It seems unlikely that the difference between general and regional anesthetics in these cases would be of great clinical significance.

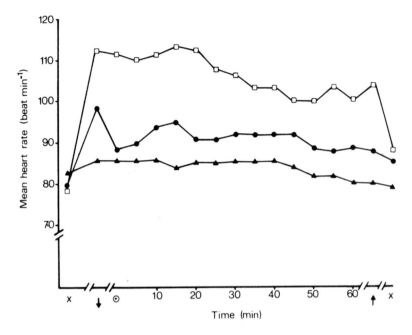

FIGURE 6–15. Mean heart rate during the course of induction, surgery, and emergence with intravenous althesin alone (open squares), althesin with spinal anesthesia (blacked circles), or althesin with fentanyl (blackened triangles). On the x-axis, xs mark the beginning and end of anesthesia, the downward arrow indicates tracheal intubation, the circle enclosing a dot indicates skin incision, and tracheal extubation is indicated by the upward arrow. *(Reproduced with permission from Blunnie et al. Br J Anaesth 55:611–618, 1983)*

HORMONAL MANIPULATION AND STRESS RESPONSE

It is possible to simulate a stress response in humans by infusing stress hormones. This "infusion-induced" stress response model has proven valuable for studying the physiologic demands created in the surgical patient.[3] There is no evidence that hormonal supplementation (such as corticosteroid use) blocks any of the precursor hormones in the stress response or alters the physiologic stress of surgery.[25] Although not a hormonal type of therapy, some adjuvants such as clonidine have been reported to decrease anesthetic utilization and oxygen consumption in the postoperative period.[26] Little other than speculation exists regarding the ability of agents targeted at the tissue level (e.g. prostaglandin inhibitors) to suppress the stress response.

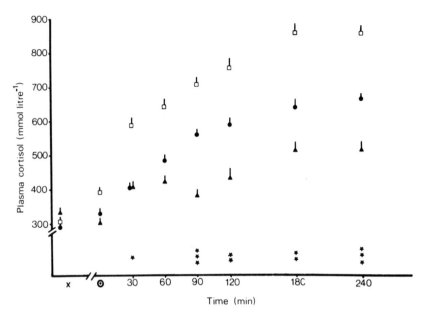

FIGURE 6–16.   Plasma cortisol levels during the course of induction, surgery, and emergence with intravenous althesin alone (open squares), althesin with spinal anesthesia (blackened circles), or althesin with fentanyl (blackened triangles). On the x-axis, an x marks the induction of anesthesia, the circle enclosing a dot indicates skin incision, and other points are indicated by time in surgery. Stars indicate differences in methods at time points reached significance at the P < .05 or better. (*Reproduced with permission from Blunnie et al. Br J Anaesth 55:611–618, 1983*)

SUMMARY OF STRESS RESPONSE

Through the use of high-dose general anesthetics or epidural and subarachnoid blocks with local anesthetics, it is possible to reduce biochemical stress markers (norepinephrine, epinephrine, and cortisol). The degree of reduction depends on many factors, including the depth of general anesthesia and the density and level of epidural or subarachnoid block.

There is no convincing evidence that peripheral nerve block or peripheral autonomic blockade significantly reduces stress response. In truly peripheral surgeries on extremities, it seems logical that interruption of neural traffic to and from the peripheral site would decrease stimulation of the central nervous system and thereby diminish the stress response. However, as stress response stimulation from

TABLE 6–6.   Comparative Degree of Changes in Plasma
Concentrations of Various Hormones or Biochemical
Measurements Used to Assess the Response to Stress After a
Standard Operation Carried Out Under Various Forms of
Anaesthesia as Defined in the Text

	Standard	Spinal	Fentanyl
Glucose	+ +	+ +	+
Cortisol	+ + +	+ + +	+
Prolactin	+ + +	+ + +	+ + +
Growth hormone	+ + +	0	+
Free fatty acids	+ + +	+ + +	+ +

Maximum percentage change from preoperative value: 0 = <20%; + = 20%–50%; + + = 50%–100%; + + + = >100%

Standard anesthesia was intravenous althesin. Spinal and fentanyl groups also had an althesin infusion. (*Reproduced with permission from Blunnie et al. Br J Anaesth 55:611–618, 1983*)

peripheral surgery is milder than that from intrathoracic or intra-abdominal surgery a clinically significant difference between general and regional anesthesia in peripheral surgeries seems unlikely. Little is known about treatments aimed at suppressing local factors such as prostanoids and kinins.

STRESS RESPONSE MODIFICATION AND OUTCOME

With expenditures for health care growing at double-digit rates and health care expenditures topping 12% of the Gross National Product in 1991, outcomes from medical expenditures are being watched closely. Cost effectiveness of anesthetics and procedures for postoperative pain control are always in question. Outcomes following surgery result from a complex interaction of preoperative, intraoperative, and postoperative factors. Recent studies have attempted to relate surgical outcomes to both biochemical and physiologic stress markers and their modification by either intraoperative anesthetic or postoperative anesthetic or analgesic interventions.[9,27–29] Table 6–7 outlines some of the characteristics and findings of these studies. Recent studies collectively suggest a relationship between intraoperative and postoperative anesthetic techniques and patient outcome.[8,9,23,30] Clearly many other variables also affect patient outcome.[31]

TABLE 6–7. Stress Response Modification and Outcome

Study/Year	Period of Intervention	Patient Population	Hypothesis	Result	Conclusion
Cuschceri/1985	postoperative N = 75	healthy adults, abdominal surgery	epidural analgesia superior	fewer postop pulmonary complications	epidural postop analgesia
Yeager/1987	intraoperative and postoperative N = 53	adult major vascular	epidural/light general superior to general alone	much reduced major organ failure	epidural/light general anesthesia protective in high risk patient
Baron/1991	intraoperative N = 173	adult major vascular	comparison of epidural/light general without control of method of postoperative pain control	no difference in major organ system failure between groups	if protective effect results from epidural, it results from postoperative use
Anand/1992	intraoperative and postoperative N = 45	pediatric congenital heart repair	opioids protective	improved survival	opioids protective in pediatric congenital heart repair
Mangano/1992	postoperative N = 106	adult coronary bypass	postoperative opioids protective in coronary bypass	• no outcome differences • No detectable hemodynamic difference • less postoperative ischemia by ECG	opioid infusion after coronary artery bypass can decrease ischemia

N = Number of patients studied

Anand and Hickey, in their recent work on opioid anesthesia in children undergoing repair of congenital heart lesions, have given some support to a link between outcome and measurable changes in .stress hormones and physiologic parameters altered by stress.[9] Yeager et al. did not show stress hormone differences between general and epidural anesthesia in the adult population they studied, but the outcome difference in their two treatment groups was large enough that the authors chose to terminate the study before reaching their intended number of study patients.[29] Mangano and colleagues have shown reduction in a physiologic stress marker (ECG documented ischemia) in a treatment group receiving prolonged postoperative opioid infusions.[27] However, Mangano et al. did not find any difference in major morbidity or mortality between treatment and control groups.[27]

In certain patient groups it appears that intraoperative anesthetic treatment, postoperative pain management, or some combination of the two can affect patient outcome. This effect seems most easily demonstrable in high-risk surgical patients with limited physiologic reserve. A need exists for further studies examining the effects of intraoperative and postoperative anesthetic manipulations on outcomes in large patient groups.

STRESS RESPONSE MODIFICATION—APPLICATION TO THE CARDIOTHORACIC SURGERY PATIENT

Patients presenting for cardiothoracic surgery span a broad spectrum of ages and diseases. Owing to disease and age demographics in the United States, the largest patient group presenting for cardiothoracic surgery consists of adults requiring coronary artery bypass grafting. Table 6–8 shows a matrix of patients presenting for cardiothoracic surgery, and Table 6–9 indicates the percentage breakdown of patients presenting at a representative tertiary referral center.*

From this table one can see that, for an intervention to significantly impact the overall morbidity and mortality for cardiothoracic patients would require either a modest affect on outcome in adult cardiac patients (72% of cases) or an astounding one in one of the other populations (28% of cases when pooled).

Table 6–10 shows data extracted from that recently published by Forrest et al., of a sample of 17,201 cases performed at multiple centers.[31] Listed are procedures requiring abdominal or thoracic incisions and the percentage of "severe" adverse cardiac and respiratory out-

TABLE 6–8.   Patients Presenting for Cardiothoracic Surgery

	Cardiovascular	Noncardiovascular
Pediatric	patent ductus arteriosus coarctation of aorta complex congenital heart lesions	tracheoesophageal fistula thoracoplasty scoliosis neoplasia flail chest bronchiectasis/abscess
Adult	coronary artery bypass heart valve replacement/repair implanted defibrillator thoracic aortic aneurysms	emphysema/bullae neoplasm flail chest bronchiectasis/abscess

TABLE 6–9.   Cardiothoracic Surgical Patients
by Procedure Type

Patient Group	Surgery Type		
	Cardiac (%)	Thoracic (%)	Total (%)
Pediatric	8	2	10
Adult	72	18	90
Total	80	20	100

comes (including death). Cardiac and respiratory adverse outcomes are responsible for the majority of morbidity and mortality. Tables 6–11 and 6–12 show the results (absolute numbers) of severe respiratory and cardiac outcomes in an operating room with 10,000 cases per year and a case distribution typical of a tertiary referral center.[31]

Note that in an operating setting such as this, although the percent of adverse outcomes is much less in group II cases, the total number of adverse outcomes is higher because of volume effects. Each 1% of change in outcome in group II would represent 48 patients versus 3 patients in Group I. What Tables 6–11 and 6–12 depict is intuitive but is often overlooked. In order to make significant overall changes in outcomes in surgical patients, one must either change outcomes slightly in large volume procedures or change outcomes by a large amount in low volume procedures.

*Bowman Gray School of Medicine/North Carolina Baptist Hospitals

TABLE 6–10. Percentage of Adverse Outcomes for Intracavitary Procedures (abdominal and thoracic)

Procedure Type	Total Procedures (%)	Severe Outcomes; Cardiac (%)	Severe Outcomes; Respiratory (%)	Total Severe Outcomes; Cardiac & Respiratory (%)
Thoracic	1	10	4	14
Cardiac	3	30	3	33
Abdominal	14	4	1	5
Gynecologic	26	5	1	6
Urologic	8	1	0.5	1.5
Column Totals	52	50	9.5	59.5

(Adapted with permission from Forrest JB, et al. Anesthesiology 72:3–15, 1992)

TABLE 6–11. Number of Severe Outcomes Per 10,000 Procedures

Case Type	Severe Cardiac Outcomes (n)	Severe Respiratory Outcomes (n)	Row Totals
Group I (Thoracic or Cardiac)	100	13	113
Group II (Abdominal, Gynecologic, and Urologic)	194	44	238
Column Totals	294	57	351

(Adapted with permission from Forrest JB et al. Anesthesiology 72:2–15, 1992)

TABLE 6–12. Sensitivity Analysis by Case Type in a Group of 10,000 Cases

Case Type	Total Procedures	Total Severe Cardiac or Respiratory Outcomes (per 10,000)	Percentage of Procedures Experiencing Severe Outcomes	Number of Severe Outcomes Represented by 1%
Group I (Thoracic or Cardiac)	300	113	28	4
Group II (Abdominal, Gynecologic, or Urological)	4800	238	4.9	49

(Adapted with permission from Forrest JB et al. Anesthesiology 72:3–15, 1992)

Adult cardiac cases represent 72% of the total cardiothoracic cases. Thirty percent of these cases have severe adverse cardiac and 3% have severe adverse respiratory outcomes. These figures may be somewhat inflated by defining an adverse outcome as something requiring medical intervention. Although not specified in the study, conceivably this might include ventricular premature beats treated with a lidocaine bolus or infusion. Slogoff and Keats have indicated there may be some relationship between perioperative ischemia related to physiologic stress (tachycardia–hypertension) and outcome in adult cardiac surgical patients.[32] Because of the reduced physiologic reserve of this group of patients prior to operative repair, it would seem that stress response suppression would be most protective if applied before repair of the heart lesion. Other periods when stress response might be beneficially modified in this group include during cardiopulmonary bypass and in the first day or two postoperatively. The use of high dose narcotics in the postoperative period could result in more pulmonary morbidity owing to the side effect of sedation.

Adult thoracic (noncardiac) procedures, the second largest group of patients presenting for cardiothoracic surgery, represent 18% of the total patients presenting for cardiothoracic surgery. Ten percent of these patients have severe adverse cardiac outcomes and 4% have severe adverse pulmonary outcomes.[31] This group has associated factors that make stress response suppression important: (1) advanced age, (2) limited cardiac reserve or coexisting cardiac disease, (3) limited pulmonary reserve or coexisting pulmonary disease, and (4) a type of incision known to compromise pulmonary function in the postoperative period. Debate about the value of postoperative stress reduction in this group of patients continues, but evidence is mounting that reduction of physiologic stress (preventing cardiopulmonary compromise) by using thoracic epidural analgesia improves outcome.[29,30] Differences in opinions about the use of thoracic epidural anesthesia in this group probably come from (1) differences in patient demographics in different studies (e.g., coexisting disease and functional impairment), (2) differences in surgical time and technique, and (3) differences in application of the epidural (skill in placement and management). As we become more proficient at managing the thoracic surgical patient at high risk both intraoperatively and postoperatively, morbidity and mortality in this group will probably improve.

Pediatric cardiac procedures represent the third largest group presenting for cardiothoracic surgery, comprising 8% of the total cardiothoracic cases. Thirty percent of pediatric cardiac patients suffer severe adverse cardiac outcomes and 3% suffer severe respiratory outcomes.[31] Anand and Hickey recently presented data concerning the use of sufentanil versus halothane, finding a significant improvement in outcome in the patients receiving sufentanil intraoperatively and postoperatively.[9] They also noted that markers of biochemical and physiologic stress were diminished in the sufentanil group. This evidence thus supports the contention that reducing intraoperative and postoperative stress in this patient population improves outcome.

Pediatric noncardiac thoracic cases are numerically the smallest group with respect to total cardiothoracic cases, compromising just 2% of the total. Severe outcomes in this group mainly consist of postoperative adverse pulmonary outcomes, possibly because of the lack of degenerative cardiac diseases commonly afflicting adults. Although reports exist about different techniques for suppressing perioperative stress (e.g., epidural and caudal blocks) in this patient group, no prospective and randomized clinical trials addressing outcome appear. Because of the relatively large physiologic reserve possessed by this group, a large series would probably be required before significant differences in outcome could be observed.

SUMMARY

In applying our knowledge about stress response reduction to cardiothoracic patients, recent studies support reducing stress response in adults undergoing noncardiac thoracic procedures by using postoperative epidural analgesia and also by reducing intraoperative and postoperative stress in pediatric cardiac patients with high dose narcotics. As both the largest number of patients and the highest complication rate occurs in adults presenting for cardiac surgery, marginal percentage gains in this group could significantly enhance patient outcomes. This group therefore offers fertile ground for future investigations about stress response suppression.

As a result of an aging society and accompanying changes in surgical disease demographics, perioperative stress reduction seems most likely to impact aged patients with preexisting cardiopulmonary disease presenting for abdominal or thoracic procedures. Large, well-controlled clinical trials will be necessary to determine which stress reduction techniques in which populations will improve outcomes in a cost-effective manner.

References

1. Cuthbertson DP: Second annual Jonathan E. Rhoads Lecture. The metabolic response to injury and its nutritional implications: Retrospect and prospect. J Par Ent Nutr 3:108–129, 1979
2. Tsuji H, Shirasaka C: Inhibition of adrenergic response to upper abdominal surgery with prolonged epidural blockade. Jpn J Surg 12:344–348, 1982
3. Bessey PQ, Watters JM, Aoki TT, Wilmore DW: Combined hormonal infusion simulates the metabolic response to injury. Ann Surg 200:264–281, 1984
4. Seitz W: Stress and the endocrine system. A contribution to the value of endocrine parameters under anesthesia and operation. Anaesth Reanim 16:147–158, 1991
5. Chwals WJ: Metabolism and nutritional frontiers in pediatric surgical patients. Assistant Professor of Surgery and Pediatrics, Division of Surgical Sciences, Department of General Surgery, Bowman Gray School of Medicine of Wake Forest University, Winston-Salem, NC 27157–1095
6. Chernow B, Alexander HR, Smallridge RC et al: Hormonal responses to graded surgical stress. Arch Intern Med 147:1273–1278, 1987
7. Roizen MF, Horrigan RW, Frazer BM: Anesthetic doses blocking adrenergic (stress) and cardiovascular responses to incision-MAC BAR. Anesthesiology 54:390–398, 1981
8. Anand KJS, Sippell WG, Aynsley-Green A: Randomised trial of fentanyl anaesthesia in preterm babies undergoing surgery: Effects on the stress response. Lancet i:62–65, 1987
9. Anand KJS, Hickey PR: Halothane–morphine compared with high-dose sufentanil for anesthesia and postoperative analgesia in neonatal cardiac surgery. N Engl J Med 326:1–9, 1992
10. Anand KJS, Ward-Platt MP: Neonatal and pediatric stress responses to anesthesia and operation. Int Anesth Clin 26:218–225, 1988
11. Crozier TA, Drobnik L, Stafforst D, Kettler D: Opiate modulation of the stress-induced increase of vasoactive intestinal peptide (VIP) in plasma. Horm Metab Res 20:352–356, 1988
12. Baron JF, Bertrand M, Barré E et al: Combined epidural and general anesthesia versus general anesthesia for abdominal aortic surgery. Anesthesiology 75:611–618, 1991
13. Delalande JP, Le Page JL, Perramant M, Lozach P, Tanguy RL: Influence of epidural anaesthesia on protein sparing in major visceral surgery. Ann Fr Anesth Réanim 3:16–21, 1954
14. Gordon NH, Scott DB, Percy-Robb IW: Modification of plasma corticosteroid concentrations during and after surgery by epidural blockade. Br Med J 1:581–583, 1973
15. Brandt MR, Fernandes A, Mordhorst R, Kehlet H: Epidural analgesia improves postoperative nitrogen balance. Br Med J 1:1106–1108, 1978
16. Brandt MR, Kehlet H, Faber O, Binder C: C-peptide and insulin during blockade of the hyperglycaemic response to surgery by epidural analgesia. Clin Endocrinol 6:167–170, 1977
17. Jorgensen BC, Andersen HB, Engquist A: Influence of epidural mor-

phine on postoperative pain, endocrine-metabolic, and renal responses to surgery. A controlled study. Acta Anesth Scand 26:63–68, 1982

18. Brandt MR, Olgaard K, Kehlet H: Epidural analgesia inhibits the renin and aldosterone response to surgery. Acta Anaesthesiol Scand 23:267–272, 1979

19. Brandt M, Kehlet H, Binder C, Hagen C, NcNeilly AS: Effect of epidural analgesia on the glycoregulatory endocrine response to surgery. Clin Endocrinol 5:107–114, 1976

20. Blunnie WP, McIlroy PDA, Merrett JD, Dundee JW: Cardiovascular and biochemical evidence of stress during major surgery associated with different techniques of anaesthesia. Br J Anaesth 55:611–618, 1983

21. Asoh T, Tsuji H, Shirasaka C, Takeuchi Y: Effects of epidural analgesia on metabolic response to major upper abdominal surgery. Acta Anaesthesiol Scand 27:233–237, 1983

22. Kehlet H: The stress response to anaesthesia and surgery: Release mechanisms and modifying factors. Clinics in Anaesthesiology 2:315–339, 1984

23. Chari P, Katariya RN, Dash RJ, Phanindranath TSN: Effect of coeliac plexus block on plasma cortisol in major abdominal surgery. Indian J Surg 42:384–387, 1980

24. Stevens RA, Artuso JD, Kao TC, Bray JG, Spitzer L, Louwsma DL: Changes in human plasma catecholamine concentrations during epidural anesthesia depend on the level of block. Anesthesiology 74:1029–1034, 1991

25. Lacoumenta S, Yeo TH, Burrin JM, Paterson JL, Hall GM: The effects of cortisol supplementation on the metabolic and hormonal response to surgery. Clin Physiol 7:455–464, 1987

26. Rademaker BMP, Sih IL, Kalkman CJ et al: Effects of interpleurally administered bupivacaine 0.5% on opioid analgesic requirements and endocrine response during and after cholecystectomy: A randomized double-blind controlled study. Acta Anaesthesiol Scand 35:108–112, 1991

27. Mangano DT, Silciano D, Hollenberg M et al: Postoperative myocardial ischemia. Therapeutic trials using intensive analgesia following surgery. The Study of Perioperative Ischemia (SPI) Research Group. Anesthesiology 76:342–353, 1992

28. Blunnie WP, McIlroy PDA, Merrett JD, Dundee JW: Cardiovascular and biochemical evidence of stress during major surgery associated with different techniques of anaesthesia. Br J Anaesth 55:611–618, 1983

29. Yeager MP, Glass DD, Neff RK, Brinck-Johnsen T: Epidural anesthesia and analgesia in high-risk surgical patients. Anesthesiology 66:729–736, 1987

30. Cuschieri RJ, Morran CG, Howie JC, McArdle CS: Postoperative pain and pulmonary complications: Comparison of three analgesic regimens. Br J Surg 72:495–498, 1985

31. Forrest JB, Rehder K, Cahalan MK, Goldsmith CH: Multicenter study of general anesthesia. III. Predictors of severe perioperative adverse outcomes. Anesthesiology 76:3–15, 1992

32. Slogoff S, Keats AS: Does perioperative myocardial ischemia lead to postoperative myocardial infarction? Anesthesiology 62:107–114, 1985

Pain Management in Cardiothoracic Surgery, edited by Gravlee and Rauck. J. B. Lippincott Company, Philadelphia © 1993.

Kyle E. Jackson

7 | Postthoracotomy Pain Syndromes

POSTTHORACOTOMY PAIN SYNDROMES

The diagnosis of Postthoracotomy Pain Syndrome (PTPS) is given to painful states in the area of the surgical incision which linger beyond the expected postoperative course. Pain following thoracotomy is generally expected to last up to 2 months. Therefore, by strict International Association for the Study of Pain (IASP) definition, the pain must persist for at last that long, even if it is severe enough to seek treatment from pain control specialists before that time.[1] Classically, PTPS is described as a sensation of continuous burning or aching in the area of the scar; although a dysesthetic or lancinating component may be present, often extending beyond the immediate area of the incision. This noxious sensation can be aggravated by such physical stimuli as pressure, touch, movement, and manipulation, as well as by temperature and emotional factors. On occasion, the movements of the shoulder girdle may intensify the pain, and resultant disuse of the upper extremity can produce a mechanically contracted shoulder joint.

Incidence

The true incidence of PTPS is difficult to assess. In one study of 126 thoracotomy patients, only 38 received any postoperative pain medications, all of which were nonnarcotic, and the remaining patients relied on nonpharmacologic means of pain control.[2] All patients reported intermittent postoperative pain in the first few days after the operation. The mean reported duration of pain was almost 7 days, with approximately 5% and 2% still experiencing pain at postoperative days 25 and 40, respectively (Fig. 7–1). From this report, one might infer that the incidence of PTPS is diminishingly small; however, more recent data suggest that the incidence is much higher than previously thought. Dajczman et al. reviewed the charts of 202 patients where at least 2 months had elapsed since their thoracotomy.[3] Of these 202 patients, 56 survivors completed a questionnaire about PTPS. The results of this survey are displayed in Table 7–1. Thirty patients had persistent pain around the incisional site. Although most had a visual analog scale (VAS) pain score of less than 4, on a scale of 1 to 10, one VAS score of seven was reported as long as 4 to

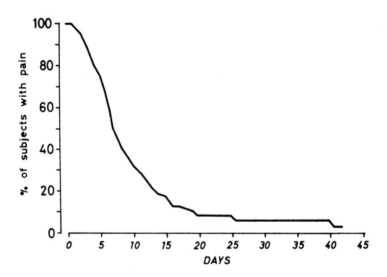

FIGURE 7–1.   An asymptotic display of patients with pain demonstrating the diminishing complaints over time. From this graph one can infer that no patient developed PTPS as no patients reached the requisite 60 days. *(Reprinted with permission from Bachiocco V et al: Funct Neurol 5:321–332, 1990)*

TABLE 7–1.

Time Postthoracotomy	Number of Patients with Pain	Total Number of Patients Evaluable	% of Evaluable Patients with Pain
<1 yr[a]	6	12	50
1–2 yrs	11	15	73
2–3 yrs	7	13	54
3–4 yrs	3	6	50
4–5 yrs	3	10	30
Total	30	56	

[a]Patients at least 2 months postthoracotomy.
(*Reprinted with permission from Dajczman E et al: Chest 99:270–274, 1991*)

5 years postoperatively. No patient reported that the pain severely interfered with their life, however some required treatment with daily analgesics, neural blockade, acupuncture, or sought relief at a multi-disciplinary pain management center.

Thus, after thoracotomies for both benign and malignant states, PTPS may occur more frequently than previously thought. Patients with PTPS seen at our pain clinic frequently display more than just the painful components evident on physical exam. They frequently have a psychological overlay to their pain syndrome. When the "cure" for a brush with cancer creates a new disease perceived to be as pernicious as the cancer, the patients may acquire depression, anxiety, desperation, and unrealistic expectations from the proposed treatment regimen. For this reason, PTPS often warrants a multidisciplinary approach. Response to treatment is often a lengthy process. Teaching coping skills through medical psychology constitutes a valuable component in maintaining the patient's outlook and hopes.

Malignant and Infectious Causes of PTPS

Thoracotomy is most commonly performed for malignancy of the lung. In 1990, lung cancer in women exceeded breast cancer as the greatest cause of cancer-related deaths (approximately 50,000 per year versus 44,000 per year), accounting for 11% of new cancers in females and nearly double that in males.[4] In addition, it causes 34% and 21% of the total cancer deaths in males and females, respectively. There were an estimated 142,000 deaths and 157,000 new cases of lung cancer in 1990, of which only 50% were considered operable.

In patients with a previous diagnosis of cancer, PTPS may result from either a benign or malignant etiology, thus recurrence of the tumor must be ruled out as the source of the pain. Kanner et al. evaluated persistent or recurrent postthoracotomy pain and its relationship to cancer in 126 patients.[5] Thirty-two of the thirty-three patients who had persistent or recurrent pain had undergone thoracotomy for malignancy, and recurrence of disease accounted for pain in 29 of these patients. In all cases, pain could be attributed to tumor or infection; and bore no relationship to either preoperative pain, postoperative chest wall involvement, or type of incision or closure. Location of the recurrent tumor was either local (16), vertebral or paravertebral (5), pleural (3), in the chest wall (3), or widespread (2). In light of this study, one can see why an exhaustive search for cancer must be performed when patients present with PTPS.

In all patients, a diagnostic work-up should start with a physical examination looking for infection as the etiology of the pain. The area of the scar should be examined for warm, swollen, erythematous skin and the area should also be palpated for fluctuance. A complete blood count and sedimentation rate can also assist in this evaluation. Although plain film X-rays with rib detail may be able to diagnose fracture as a cause of pain, they are insufficient to rule out metastatic disease. A CT scan and/or MRI of the chest are indispensable in trying to ascertain the presence of tumor and may help guide the pain treatment plan. In addition, a bone scan may be helpful to assess the possibility of bony metastases.

Treatment

Treatment of metastatic-related thoracotomy pain should begin in a comprehensive and step-wise fashion (Fig. 7–2). This should include an initial assessment of the likely source and quality of the pain. Classification of pain with respect to its clinical characteristics and pathogenesis represents a recent focus in chronic pain management. Arnér & Arnér published what may be a landmark article in evaluating the source and characterizing the pain as either somatic, visceral, continuous, intermittent, or neurogenic.[6] They also assessed the efficacy of epidural narcotics in treatment of these subsets of pain types. They found that patients having *continuous* somatic or visceral pain were more likely to obtain pain relief from epidural morphine than were patients experiencing *intermittent* somatic or visceral pains. Nonetheless, intermittent pain responded better to epidural narcotics than did

Cancer Pain Management

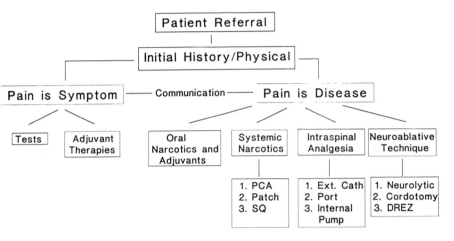

FIGURE 7–2. A useful algorithm for management of cancer related pain. Treatment generally progresses from left to right, however, in certain cases one may start with neuroablative techniques.

either neurogenic pain or pain from cutaneous sources such as cancerous ulcers or fistulae. This concept of classification of cancer pain by its response to spinal narcotics and adjuncts has been discussed by others and applies to PTPS.[7,8]

Early in its presentation, most non-neurogenic cancer-related pains respond to oral medications. Nonsteroidal anti-inflammatory agents with or without low potency oral narcotics may satisfactorily treat these patients. One should remember to dose the narcotic medication on a fixed schedule and not on a "prn" basis. This type of therapy has been shown to more effectively sustain analgesic levels of pain medication. Also, the anxiety experienced by cancer patients who take medication whenever the pain recurs is diminished when the medications are taken on a scheduled basis.[9]

If the pain is not relieved by these low potency medications, the possibility of treating the disease with additional chemotherapy, surgery, or radiation therapy should be evaluated. Once these modalities are exhausted, then the cancer pain should be treated as the primary disease (Fig. 7–2). If the more potent narcotics are not helpful, either the doses are inadequate or the pain is poorly responsive to narcotics. If eliciting a careful history indicates that narcotics reduce the pain temporarily, the physician should increase the dose, decrease the dosing interval, or perhaps both. Narcotics should be liberally increased until the patient either becomes comfortable or acquires intolerable nausea and vomiting or sedation. If intolerable side effects are reached before the quality of pain relief is maximized, spinal narcotics should be strongly considered. Epidural or intrathecal narcotics achieve greater analgesia at a given dose, and thus may allow better control of pain than the oral, intravenous, or subcutaneous routes. Once pain control is achieved, increasing the dose and basal infusion may eventually become necessary as a result of tolerance or increasing tumor burden.

Certain malignant pain syndromes cannot be adequately treated by spinal narcotics alone. Neurogenic pain, as noted by neurologic involvement on diagnostic imaging, or inferred from the quality of pain complaints often requires an adjuvant such as the antiepileptic carbamazepine in addition to spinal narcotics. The proposed mechanism of pain relief is thought to involve frequency-dependent inhibition of sodium channels.[10] Tonicly active A-delta and C-fibers mediating neurogenic pain would be more sensitive to this effect than more quiescent nerves. Other adjuvant medications that may be used on neurogenic pain include valproic acid, mexiletine, and dilantin. If the patient responds incompletely despite the adjuvant medications, one may consider the addition of local anesthetic to the narcotic administered through the epidural or spinal catheter.[8] In patients who have persistent pain despite applying these treatment options, neuroablative procedures (e.g. epidural phenol) should be considered. Newer agents such as epidural clonidine may play an increased role in treatment of these recalcitrant malignant pain syndromes.[11]

Benign Causes of PTPS

PTPS from nonmalignant etiologies may also have multiple components and thus the patient may require more than one treatment modality. Classically, most benign forms of PTPS are thought to be neurogenic. Benign neurogenic pains are not unique to thoracotomies, and may be seen in many other postsurgical states.[12,13,14]

The healing pattern of the scar does not predict PTPS.[12] Well healed, normal appearing scars may be just as painful as scars with keloid formation. Typical neurogenic pain may have a dysesthetic quality on light touch, as well as a continuous burning, aching component in a distribution extending beyond the scar. Demyelination of nerve fibers is implicated in the pain. Subsequent impulse transmission through large previously myelinated fibers may cross over to smaller nonmyelinated nerve fibers that transmit pain. Alternatively, compression neuropathy may preferentially damage large fibers, and the resulting imbalance between large and small fibers may facilitate transmission of noxious impulses.

Treatment

Intercostal neuralgias extending beyond the scar can be both diagnosed and treated by local anesthetic application via intercostal nerve block. Some evidence suggests that the addition of a corticosteroid to the local anesthetic may reduce the pain; especially if the pain character implies that C-fibers may be involved (aching, burning types of pain).[15] A series of intercostal nerve blocks may gradually decrease the pain. Posterolateral thoracotomy incisions are often made at upper thoracic levels, and this can be difficult to anesthetize with intercostal nerve blocks because the scapula obscures distinct palpation of the ribs. For this reason, one should consider thoracic epidural anesthesia to treat pain syndromes that extend into the upper thoracic regions. Some clinicians have proposed that sympathetic blockade may have some benefit in or treatment of painful peripheral nerve syndromes.[16] One may infer that paravertebral blocks would be helpful because neural blockade, more proximally than intercostal nerve blocks, would also anesthetize sympathetic fibers. However, the use of contrast medium mixed with local anesthetics was shown with computed tomography to frequently spread into the epidural space, which would thus produce a sympathetic block.[17] The author believes that the risk of pneumothorax with paravertebral blocks would render thoracic epidural anesthesia a more desirable treatment option. As with malignant neurogenic pains, the addition of an antiepileptic drug may reduce the pain.

Some propose cryoanalgesia as a method to induce long-term analgesia in this pain syndrome. Cryoanalgesia involves freezing the nerve so that an ice ball reaching temperatures of $-20°C$ surrounds the nerve. The resultant axonal degeneration and breakdown of the myelin results in temporary neural blockade. The presence of intact endoneurium allows axonal regeneration and subsequent return of sensation. Early studies demonstrated that both freezing cycles greater than 30 seconds and application of more than one freezing cycle resulted in excessive cutaneous numbness.[18] More recent data suggests that a single freeze cycle under 30 seconds is most appropriate.[19] Caution should be applied in performing intercostal cryoanalgesia above the T5 dermatome in women, as this may lead to an unpleasant sensation in the area of the breast. Although some concern might arise about exacerbating the neuralgic pain with this reversibly neurodestructive treatment option, other authors have not shown neurologic injury to be a problem with cryoanalgesia.[20] These data were reported in use of cryoanalgesia for postoperative thoracotomy pain, and specific data evaluating its role in PTPS is lacking. Preliminary data show that cryoanalgesia performed at the time of thoracotomy may be more efficacious than either epidural narcotics or interpleural analgesia in preventing PTPS.[21] However, these data also need confirmation with a larger series of patients.

When a postsurgical neuroma can be discreetly localized within the scar, very small amounts (<1 ml) of local anesthetic should be placed on the neuroma.[22] If this approach relieves the pain, the procedure may be repeated with the same volume of a neurolytic phenol solution. This has been shown to produce a remarkably long-lasting benefit, although it may be necessary to repeat the block if a single injection incompletely relieves the pain. Smaller unmyelinated fibers are most susceptible to the neurodestructive action of carbolic acid (phenol), however the total effect to the nerve depends on the concentration and volume of the agent. A painful peripheral neuritis may develop when such a procedure is performed more proximally with intent to destroy the entire peripheral nerve, thus the distinction between neurolytic blockade of a small peripheral neuroma versus neurolysis of the entire intercostal nerve cannot be overemphasized.

Capsaician, a substance derived from the plant *capsicum*, has been shown to have the following effects:[23]

1. Initially it stimulates afferent C-fibers and causes transmitter release at peripheral nerve terminals
2. Repeat doses cause a sensory blockade of capsaician sensitive fibers through inhibition of neuronal impulse propagation.
3. Sustained use depletes the releasable pool of neurotransmitters.

When applied to dysesthetic, painful skin, this ointment proves beneficial in syndromes similar to PTPS.[24] One must inform patients that the initial application of capsaician may increase their burning pain, but this side effect should abate with subsequent applications.[25]

Musculoskeletal Causes

Although PTPS most commonly involves neurogenic pain, a muscular etiology may be superimposed on the previously cited causes of pain. For years, thoracotomy by posterolateral incision had been the standard for exposure of the mediastinum, hilum, and lung. This incision may split the latissimus dorsi, trapezius, rhomboid major, and serratus anterior muscles. Studies have shown that the surgical incision may have a relationship not only to postoperative pulmonary function, but also to the severity of postoperative pain.[26,27] The lateral limited thoracotomy, by dividing the serratus anterior in the line of its fibers and by mobilizing the latissimus dorsi without dividing it, may avoid some of this trauma.[28] This incision would allow a better postoperative use of the shoulder, thus preventing a restricted range of motion (Fig. 7–3). The physical examination should include pal-

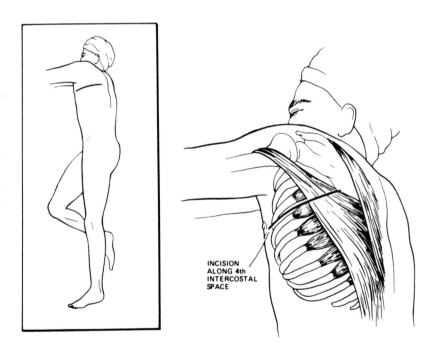

INCISION
ALONG 4th
INTERCOSTAL
SPACE

FIGURE 7–3.   The lateral limited thoracotomy along the 4th intercostal space. Note that the more medial portion of the incision does not transect the latissimus dorsi but is beneath this muscle after it is mobilized. *(Reprinted wtih permission from Mitchell RL et al: J Thorac Cardiovasc Surg 99;590–596, 1990)*

pation searching for painful musculature along the side of the thorax, upper back, and shoulder, as well as restricted range of motion of the shoulder girdle.

A specific type of musculoskeletal PTPS can be categorized as myofascial pain syndromes (MPS). This disorder consists of distinct, localized areas originating in muscles which, when palpated, cause reproducible pain referred to distance areas. In PTPS, the most common MPS seen would probably be located in the serratus anterior, latissimus dorsi, or rhomboid muscles.[29]

Treatment

Both MPS and painful impaired range of motion in the shoulder respond best to a combination of treatment modalities, of which physical therapy techniques represent mainstays. Stretching, strengthening, and increasing tone may not only reduce the pain but also improve mobilization. Adjuvant techniques such as heat, massage, ultrasound, iontophoresis, phonophoresis and vapocoolant spray with stretching may improve patient compliance and efficacy. Often trigger point injections can relieve pain and facilitate physical therapy. Pharmacologic intervention may also improve the symptoms of MPS. One should consider NSAIDs, as well as muscle relaxants (e.g., cyclobenzaprine, methocarbamol) to treat presumed inflammatory pain or muscle spasm. If the patient's sleep is impaired, low dose tricyclic antidepressants (TCAs) may also be added. TCAs not only improve sleep, but have been shown to decrease patients' perception of pain independent of their antidepressant effect.[30] Some also advocate the use of Transcutaneous Electrical Nerve Stimulation (TENS) to treat myofascial pain syndromes. Because the risk of TENS is virtually negligible, one should have a low threshold for prescribing a trial of this modality. Narcotics have almost no role in treatment of MPS, and their use should be discouraged because addiction may result.

SUMMARY

Postthoracotomy pain syndrome has multiple etiologies. Although the treatment modalities overlap somewhat, the most effective therapy results when one has a working diagnosis of the probable pain mechanism. Physical diagnosis and diagnostic imaging are crucial to distinguishing a malignant versus a nonmalignant etiology, so this should constitute the initial diagnostic focus. Neural blockade need not be the primary focus in treatment of postthoracotomy pain syndromes, as a combination of noninvasive treatments often alleviates the patient's complaint. Both local anesthetics and neurolytic agents may be appropriate for some postthoracotomy pain syndromes. However, a clear understanding of the potential risk and benefit of these procedures must be understood by both the physician and the patient. In the future, prospective studies are needed not only to identify the true incidence of postthoracotomy pain syndromes, but also to compare the efficacies of different treatment options for this recalcitrant pain syndrome.

References

1. Post-thoracotomy pain syndrome (XVII–14) Classification of chronic pain. Pain Suppl 3:S138, 1986
2. Bachiocco V, Morselli-Labate AM, Rusticali AG, Bragaglia R, Mastrorilli M, Carli GC: Intensity, latency and duration of post-thoracotomy pain: Relationship to personality traits. Func Neurol 5(4):321–332, 1990
3. Dajczman E, Gordon A, Kreisman H, Wolkove N: Long-term post-thoracotomy pain. Chest 99:270–274, 1991
4. Scanlon EF: Breast cancer. In Holleb HI, Furk DJ, Murphy GP (eds): American Cancer Society Textbook of Clinical Oncology, pp. 177–193. Atlanta, GA, American Cancer Society, 1991
5. Kanner RM, Martini N, Foley KM: Nature and incidence of post-thoracotomy pain. Proc Am Soc Clin Oncol Abstr C–590, 1982
6. Arnér S, Arnér B: Differential effects of epidural morphine in the treatment of cancer-related pain. Acta Anaesthesiol Scand 29:32–36, 1985
7. Sjöberg M, Appelgren L, Einarsson S, Huttman E, Linder LE, Nitescu P, Curelaru I: Long-term intrathecal morphine and bupivicaine in "refractory" cancer pain. I. Results from the first series of 52 patients. Acta Anaesthesiol Scand 35:30–43, 1991
8. Samuelsson H, Hedner T: Pain characterization in cancer patients and the analgetic responses to epidural morphine. Pain 46:3–8, 1991
9. Ferrer-Brechner T: Practical management of pain. In Raj P (ed): Rationale Management of Cancer Related Pain, p. 312–328. Yearbook Medical Publishers, Inc., 1986
10. Tanelian DL, Brose WG: Neuropathic pain can be relieved by drugs that are use-dependent sodium channel blockers: Lidocaine, carbamazepine, and mexiletine. Anesthesiology 74:949–951, 1991
11. Eisenach JC, Rauck RL, Buzzanell C, Lysak SZ: Epidural clonidine analgesia for intractable cancer pain: Phase I, Anesthesiology 71:647–652, 1989
12. Carlsson CA, Persson K, Pelletieri L: Painful scars after thoracic and abdominal surgery. Acta Chir Scand 151:309–311, 1985

13. Defalque RJ, Bromley JJO: Poststernotomy neuralgia: A new pain syndrome. Anesth Analg 69:81–82, 1989
14. Vecht CJ, VandeBrand HJ, Wajer OJM: Post-axillary dissection pain in breast cancer due to a lesion of the intercostal brachial nerve. Pain 38:171–176, 1989
15. Johansson A, Hao J, Sjolund B: Local corticosteroid application blocks transmission in normal nociceptive C-fibers. Acta Anaesthesiol Scand 34:335–338, 1990
16. Bennett GJ: Guest editorial: The role of the sympathetic nervous system in painful peripheral neuropathy. Pain 45:221–223, 1991
17. Purcell-Jones G, Pither CE, Justins DM: Paravertebral somatic nerve block: A clinical, radiographic, and computed tomographic study in chronic pain patients. Anesth Analg 68:32–39, 1989
18. Glynn CJ, Lloyd JW, Barnard JDW: Cryoanalgesia in the management of pain after thoracotomy. Thorax 35:325–327, 1980
19. Maiwand MO, Makey AR, Rees A: Cryoanalgesia after thoracotomy: Improvement of technique and review of 600 cases. J Thorac Cardiovasc Surg 92:291–295, 1986
20. Johannesen N, Madsen G, Ahlburg P: Neurological sequelae after cryoanalgesia for thoracotomy pain relief. Ann Chir Gynaecol 79:108–109, 1990
21. Miguel R, Hubbell D: Does the postoperative pain relieving technique affect the incidence of postthoracotomy pain syndrome? ASA Abstr, Anes 75:A763, 1991
22. Kirvella O, Nieminen S: Treatment of painful neuromas with neurolytic blockade. Pain 41:161–165, 1990
23. Lembeck F, Donner J: The wide spectrum of functions of capsaician—Sensitive nociceptive afferents. In Sicuteri Fetal (eds): Advances in Pain Research and Therapy, vol. 20. New York, Raven Press, 1992
24. Watson CPN, Evans RJ, Watt VR: The post-masectomy pain syndrome and the effect of topical capsaician. Pain 38:177–186, 1989
25. Fusco BM, Alessandri M: Analgesic effect of capsaicin in idiopathic trigeminal neuralgia. Anesth Analg 74:375–377, 1992
26. Lemmer J, Gomez MN, Symreng T, Ross AF, Ross NP: Limited lateral thoracotomy improved postoperative pulmonary function, Arch Surgery 125:873–877, 1990
27. Hazelrigg SR, Landreneau RJ, Boley TM: The effect of muscle-sparing versus standard posterior lateral thoracotomy on pulmonary function, muscle strength, and postoperative pain. J Thorac Cardiovasc Surg 101:394–401, 1991
28. Mitchell RL: The lateral limited thoracotomy incision: Standard for pulmonary operations. J Thorac Cardiovasc Surg 99:590–596, 1990
29. Travell JG, Simmons DG: Myofacial and Pain Dysfunction: The Trigger Point Manual, Serratus Anterior Muscle "Stitch-in-the-Side," pp. 622–629. Baltimore, MD, Williams & Wilkins, 1983
30. Max MB, Kishore-Kumar R, Schafer SC, Meister B, Gracely RH, Smoller B, Dubner R: Efficacy of desipramine in painful diabetic neuropathy: A placebo-controlled trial. Pain 45:3–9, 1991

Index

Page numbers followed by (*t*) indicate tables; page numbers followed by (*f*) indicate figures.

ISBN 0-397-51293-7

90000

9 780397 512935